The Making of a Wonderful Life

Albanian Attachment

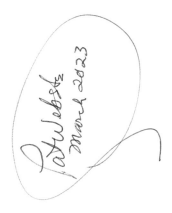

Cherie Y. Mullins

ISBN 978-1-0980-1598-5 (paperback)
ISBN 978-1-0980-1599-2 (digital)

Copyright © 2020 by Cherie Y. Mullins

All rights reserved. No part of this publication may be reproduced, distributed, or transmitted in any form or by any means, including photocopying, recording, or other electronic or mechanical methods without the prior written permission of the publisher. For permission requests, solicit the publisher via the address below.

Christian Faith Publishing, Inc.
832 Park Avenue
Meadville, PA 16335
www.christianfaithpublishing.com

Cover Photo created by: Kerri Mullins

Printed in the United States of America

Contents

Foreword 9
Preface 11
Acknowledgments 13
Prologue 21
A Very Brave Missionary 25
The Making of a Wonderful Life "Albanian Attachment" 50
Roger's Calling to Albania 55
Early Memories 61
The Tag Center: Trek For Hope 2000 65
Those Howard Boys 80
This I Believe 87
Albania: The Next Step 93
Cherie's First Trip to Albania 102
Tirana Orphanage 114
Getting to Know the Albanian People 118
First Meeting with the Albanian Government 121
A Hole in Her Heart 128
First Granddaughter 130
A Great Missionary and Friend, David Hosaflook 138
First Assignment with Hope For the World 147
Theresa Weaver 149
A Slumber Party to Remember 159
Alketa: A First Employee 163
Second Granddaughter 165
Marga: An Orphan's Story 170

Viola's Amazing Blessing	183
Andi Demcellari	188
Etleva's Miracle	191
Mentoring at Home	199
Ikim! Ikim! Let's Get Out of Here!	209
Kosovo War Memories	212
Meet The Zefi Family	219
In Prenda's Own Words	219
Fredi's Testimony	223
From Mirela's Heart	228
Caught in a Blood Revenge	235
Albanian Adoptions	239
Rozana's Story	240
Miracle of "Night of Hope"	243
The Hope Center	248
Pam Arney, Called By God	255
Activities at the Home Office	260
Cindy's Comments	273
Staff Testimonies	281
Margarita Gjoni	281
Teuta Korra	283
Albana Lika	284
Nikolin Lekaj	286
Ledina's Story	287
Our Work in Saranda	298
Fatos's Testimony	301
Mirela's Testimony	303
Buddy's Thoughts	306
Kerri Says	312
Roger's Reflections	316
Roger's Double Whammy	323
Muddy Water Boys	328
Hope for the World Community Church Becomes a Reality	331
Come with Us	340
Epilogue: Israel	343

Reader's Remarks

I have had the wonderful blessing of seeing firsthand what the Mullins through Hope for the World have done for the beautiful country and precious people of Albania. Their passion is love in action! Their story is inspirational! Their commitment is a testimony of God's love!

—Gwen Creasman

What a great joy it was to read your book, *The Making of a Wonderful Life: Joyous Journey* and get that "backside" of your journey. You did such a great job in telling the story and I commend you for it. I hope the book will have a wide circulation.

—Evangelist "Junior" Hill

My life has truly been blessed by having read your book, *The Making of a Wonderful Life: Joyous Journey*. This book was everything I believe a book should be to the reader. I found myself laughing, crying, feeling proud for your family, and growing spiritually. I have a special place in my heart for you and your family for having read your story.

—Lucy Hopson

"I have read all three of Cherie Mullins' books. Cherie is a great writer and excellent story teller. Each one of her books contains honest and inspiring stories about how God gave her and her family the strength needed to face the challenges life brings and how He provided for them through all of their years in ministry. On each occasion she and her family persevered through various trials and still managed to continue to joyfully spread the Good News, serving the Lord through evangelism and gospel music. I think her family's life story reflects how true meaning in life awaits those who faithfully serve the Lord."

—Alex Jones

Cherie's books allow us a glimpse into a life overflowing with testimony to God's faithfulness to keep His promises. They leave us smiling as they remind us of some of our own dear memories and they challenge us to acknowledge the same faithful love and care of God towards us in our own lives. They are more evidence that loving and serving God really is the foundation of a wonderful life.

—Reda Adams

Books written by Cherie Mullins are so special because she speaks from her heart when she writes and that makes it so personal. I feel that is what draws people to what she is writing. It's like we are sitting down in her living room listening to her speak.

—Pamelia Godfrey

To all of the orphans in Albania who we have had the privilege of working with since 1992, when Hope for the World's leadership first set foot in your country. You may not realize it, but it is because of you that we were invited to come to Albania and to bring "our God," the God of the Bible, to your country.

Many of you are now in your adult lives. You are married with children of your own. You are a great tribute to your society because of wonderful things you learned while in the orphanages of Albania and through education, guidance, discipline, activities, and the love shown to you through Hope for the World and their staff.

Many of you have been fortunate enough to spend your high school years at the Hope Center in Marikaj, Albania, where you have learned so many life lessons. Your *hearts were captured* by the love of Christ there. Your *minds were challenged* through the academic mentorship and assistance so that you went on to further your education in the universities. Some of you have had specific vocational training to ensure that you have a good job and are able to support yourself and your own family. But many of you can say, *your lives were changed* because Hope for the World and its staff took time to love you and teach you some very valuable life lessons from the Word of God.

It may take you a while to appreciate fully the blessing it was for you to grow up in a government home that allowed Hope for the World to be a part of your lives. Although your families may have had no choice but to put you in a government institution, God had his plans for you, and you were not abandoned nor forgotten by him. We are thrilled that he chose us to come alongside and be an encouragement.

As the wife of Roger Mullins, the American Director of Hope for the World in Albania, it has been a tremendous privilege to get to know you. In our office in America, our daughter, Cindy, and Roger and I love seeing your photos, reading your life stories, and watching you grow. Many families, individuals, and churches have been contributing sacrificially for years to give you a better quality of life. I thank you on their behalf as well for the lovely pictures you have colored, the many thank you notes you have written and the prayers you have prayed. Best of all has been the opportunity many have had to come to Albania and experience your hugs and kisses and thank yous in person.

May the God of the Bible bless you in years to come. May he give you long life, good health, and strength of character to overcome whatever life brings your way. I wish you success in all that you do because you are indeed "A Child of the Father." You, children, are the "key" to the door that opened for Hope for the World to enter Albania.

With much love and many prayers, Gjyshe Cherie.

Foreword

I am honored that Cherie would ask me to write this foreword to her latest book. I have known Cherie and Roger and their amazing family, for over thirty-five years. As I look back over these years and think about my greatest and most memorable experiences in the ministry, Cherie and her husband Roger were there. Cherie received her salvation in a moment, but it did not end there. She refused to settle for just living the Christian life "on the surface." Her life has been an adventure of faith, ministry, and unbelievable challenges that reveal God is always at work behind the scenes, that his grace is sufficient, and that he is always faithful. I love the way Cherie and the Holy Spirit partner together to inspire us with their warm and genuine way of revealing God in the challenges and adventures that accompanied their many years of ministry to the orphans of Albania.

Cherie is a wife, mother, grandmother, and now a great-grandmother. She is a musician, songwriter, singer, speaker, and author, all while travelling the United States and the world alongside her husband in evangelism and missions. When Hope for the World was in desperate need of a director for Albania, Roger and Cherie answered that call. Since 1994, along with their outstanding Albanian staff, they have led the ministry of Hope for the World. The Albanian government has recognized this mission as the number one NGO (nongovernmental organization) in the nation.

Some authors aim for the mind, others for the heart, and a few for the soul. With this, her latest book, *Albanian Attachment*, Cherie Mullins touches all three. She shows us how to connect with God in times of great need and to celebrate God in times of great blessings. She shows us when we cannot trace the hand of God to trust the heart of God in the countless challenges, twists, and turns on their journey. In this book, Cherie convinces us that God leads a step at a time and God provides a day at a time as she draws from their experiences working in the ministry of Hope for the World in Albania since 1994.

Too often, we read a book that clinically analyzes the subject but fails to connect our hearts to God. In this book, Cherie brings us into the throne room of God. I pray this collection of amazing stories of real-life experiences and personal testimonies will encourage and inspire you on your own journey of faith to receive and recognize the blessings of God. I know that after reading this book, you will experience a stronger faith, and you will be more confident in his power.

Jimmy Franks, Founder
Hope for the World
www.HFTW.org

Preface

To those of you who have read my previous book subtitled *Joyous Journey*, you will recall that the last chapter was taken from my daily journal of a mission trip to the country of Romania. At the time when we went to Romania, Roger and I had no idea that we would ever be called by God to be missionaries to a foreign country anywhere. We both just felt that it was another "mission trip" for us and once it was over, we would pretty much go back to life in the "land of familiar."

What was familiar to us? Singing and preaching the gospel from church to church, encouraging the saints, and asking God to bring precious souls to a saving knowledge of Christ through our efforts. We have always *loved* foreign missions, and, as a family, we had met many missionaries through the years and were even supporting a number of them from our ministry. In a way, when you added all of that together and threw in a few mission trips from time to time, I guess we may have felt that we were doing our part in global missions.

As a matter of fact, since Roger was an evangelist for so many years, it had been his privilege to make wonderful friendships with many pastors, and he spent quality time with them in their offices. He was told over and over again by many pastors that there was hardly a day that went by that he didn't receive a call from some missionary, or candidate to be a missionary, asking for an opportunity to come to the church and present their ministry and ask the church to support them financially.

Roger would say to himself, and sometimes to me, "I sure am glad I'm not a missionary!" (because it's tough for them to get into many churches to raise the personal support to get them on the field). His heart would literally break for the missionaries, but at the same time, he was happy we were in the field of evangelism, where churches were calling and inviting us to come, rather than the other way around. We were blessed in that we did have a lot of invitations during our evangelism years largely because we were able to furnish not only the preacher for the revival but also the special music. This was very appealing to churches, a sort of "two-for-one" deal. We were very grateful for the many churches that invited us to come and were always amazed and honored when they would ask us to come back again and again. Another thing that was especially attractive to the churches about our family was that we brought our own housing. Our bus served as our home in every way except when it came to IRS deductions. They wouldn't allow bus repairs as "home improvements."

That being said, God has a great way of humbling us and turning things completely around in order to fulfill his perfect will and plan; at least he did so in our lives.

This particular book, which I am calling *Albanian Attachment*, is one I want to share with you to help you understand the many ways in which God changed our ministry and made us switch gears and go in a very different direction from the one in which we had been traveling. The work in Albania is mission work, but in every way, it has become a real *attachment* to our lives, to us as individuals, and even to our family members.

In many ways, these years since 1994 have been the most fulfilling and satisfying years of our lives, but in other ways, they have also been the most challenging. I hope that the next pages will reveal to you exactly what I mean by that statement.

Acknowledgments

I have found that this book has truly been a book of many combined efforts. It has taken me longer to put this book together than any of the others in my series. My very first little book was a special one that I wrote accompanying a musical project recorded by our family entitled "A Wonderful Life". I used the title of that song to springboard my booklet I wrote at that time, entitled simply, "The Making of a Wonderful Life," referring specifically to the making of that particular project. There was a song recorded by my husband on that project entitled "I've Had a Wonderful Life," When we heard that song for the first time, it seemed so very fitting for our family. Roger actually adopted it as his own testimony song. I put a little subtitle under the title to that particular book to sort of describe its contents. The subtitle is *Recording Reflections*. That was in 1997, and I had no idea that I would ever be writing another book.

For some reason, after a number of years had passed by, I began to feel compelled to write a book that would be sort of a salute to my Christian heritage. It seemed that the older I got, the more I appreciated my parents, my grandparents, yes, and even my great-grandparents. I wanted to preserve some of the great stories from our family's background so that my own children, grandchildren, and great-grandchildren could connect to their deep roots and family traditions. I wanted to share with them many of the stories I had been telling them through the years, and they had actually begged me to write. So that book came to fruition and was published in 2011, entitled *The Making of a Wonderful Life*, subtitled *Family Foundations*. That book covered my earliest years that I could remember, up until

Roger and I were married, had the two children, and were getting ready to enter Bible college.

It seemed to me that I was sort of "on a roll" so to speak with my writing by then. I felt God nudging me to keep going with these life stories as we seemed to have three distinct seasons of ministry as a family. We had the church staff ministry, evangelism years, and, finally, missions. I felt like I needed to pick up from Family Foundations and write a book to encompass the years we spent on church staffs and then on the road in evangelism and gospel music. I had no idea how big a book that would be, but I finished it and published it in 2014. It carries the same name, *The Making of a Wonderful Life*, subtitled *Joyous Journey*.

I knew from the very beginning that I would have to write a book about our ministry that has taken place during our senior years as missionaries with Hope for the World in the country of Albania. This particular book has taken me about four years to complete.

This has been my most difficult book to put together because I have included so many of our wonderful staff, missionaries, and friends who have been connected with us and our ministry in Albania. I am so grateful to each one of them for being willing to write their testimonies. And once again, I am so very thankful for my editor, Pam Godfrey, for the awesome job she did once more in editing for me. She is a lifelong friend and very good at what she does. She keeps me smiling (laughing out loud really), and she and her husband, Terry, accompanied us in September of 2018 to Albania. We made more memories we will never forget. Thank you, Pam, for your help and encouragement.

I need to thank so many for their help in getting this story told. I want to say a big personal thank you to a wonderful missionary friend, Gesina Blaauw, from the Netherlands, whose story you will enjoy in the first pages. She knew our founder, Jimmy Franks, personally, and it was through his contact with her that we came to know her as well. She was so kind to share her story with me and allow me to include it within the pages of *Albanian Attachment*. You are a wonderful blessing and inspiration to many. You were also a great friend in allowing us to purchase our Hope Center property in

Marikaj from you when you moved part of your ministry to another country. We will never forget you and the way you let God use you to help us in this matter.

Brother Jimmy Franks and his wife, Janice, have been personal friends of ours since way back in our evangelism years in the 1980s. It was because of him that Roger made his first trip to Albania. We want to thank him so much for helping the Lord direct us to our next step in ministry after Roger retired from his years on the road in evangelism and gospel music. We could not have had a ministry in Albania without you. Like Aaron was to Moses, so have you been to Roger, holding up his arms. Thank you is not at all enough for us to say. You have continued to be here with us, visiting Albania many times and supporting the work faithfully all of these past twenty-five years (as of 2019).

I wish to thank you also for your contribution to this book. You set the foundation in Albania for a great work that is still going and growing.

To Perparim Demcellari, who has been our Albanian in-country president for the past twenty years, there are not enough words or space to write all of the many ways in which you are appreciated. We love and thank you not only for what you have written in this book but mainly for the huge effect you have had on the ministry of Hope for the World in Albania since we met so many years ago. You and Aferdita have had a great impact on our ministry. Without your strong leadership and integrity, Hope for the World would not have been as highly respected by the government as it is today. Your work with us and our staff has been amazing. You have also stretched the mission dollars to impossible limits many times. God has used you in more ways than we can name.

I would also like to say a special big personal thank you for the part you have had in this book. You are such an encouragement, and I appreciate all that you did to inspire me to write of our years in your wonderful country. We love our life here on earth with you, and we look so forward to eternity in heaven together as well. I also include in my thanks to you, a very special thank you to your children, Viola and Andi, for their thoughtful remarks. Your whole family, being some of the first believers in Albania, has proven faithful all these years.

To Fred Tag, whose story you will enjoy about his awesome bike ride across America for the orphans, I thank you for your time helping me with this book and for telling your story. Thanks also for the photos. You have been a great blessing to our ministry through the years. You and your wife, Debbie, have been wonderful sponsors and have visited Albania a number of times. You have also encouraged your daughter, Heather, to make several mission trips to Albania, and she has blessed the orphans with her music and her sweet spirit of service to the Lord. We can never repay you for that long "Trek for Hope" you made in 2000.

To another great friend and missionary, David Hosaflook, I want to let you know that I appreciate you for allowing me to interview you for my book. We are very blessed by your life's work in Albania. You and Kristi and family have played a great part in the salvation and discipleship of our staff members in Shkodra, Albania. We hesitate to think where our own ministry would be without your godly influence. Thank you for taking the time to contribute to this book, and thank you for your dedicated service to the Lord in Albania.

I wish to combine three wonderful staff workers from Shkoder in this particular acknowledgement. The very first employees, Mirela and Alketa, and then later on, Etleva. Each of you has written your testimony for my book, and you have each been a great blessing in my life personally and in the lives of so many orphan children in Albania. Thank you so much for all you have done to assist me in putting this book together. I am so blessed to call each one of you my friend. Your lives have been and will continue to be a living testimony for Christ.

Next is Marga, a true orphan girl, who never knew of a mother or father, I want to thank you so much for opening your heart and bringing out some hurtful past memories to include in your testimony. I do not take that for granted. I appreciate you and love the blessing that God has given you in your marriage to our friend, Tony Waters. It's also so great to be fellow church members with you two. We never get tired of spending time with you.

I am so very grateful for the lives and testimonies of two very special people, Fredi and Prenda Zefi. Prenda and Fredi came to our organization as single young people. God put them together, and now they bless so many touching the lives of babies, children, and even adults in their work with Hope for the World and their own local church.

You are such a blessing to me personally, Fredi and Prenda. I love to be called Mother by both of you and Grammy by your children. God has truly knit our hearts together through the years since we have had you in our employ since 2000. Thanks to each of you for writing a portion of your testimonies for my book. Thank you for opening your home to our family and so many friends from America. But thank you the most for loving the orphan children. You are not only raising your own children but so many, many who would not know the love of family if it was not for you. Thank you for bringing those orphans into your home and showing them the true love found in a Christ-centered home.

Pam Arney, my heart of thanks and love goes to you for the wonderful job you not only did for this book but that you are doing daily at the Hope Center in Albania with our teens. Thank you for being such an integral part in their lives every day and night. Also for your great help in the new church and the community children's Bible classes, I thank you. Your longevity in Albania proves you are truly a God-called missionary. Thanks so much, Pam. Roger and I love you, and we love that when you come home to the states, it is to "Georgia," where we also live.

To Ledina Rabdishta, what could we do without you? You have written a great chapter in my book, and I appreciate it so very much. The day that God allowed Perparim to hire you as his next administrative assistant, when Anila married an American and moved here, was truly a great day for Hope for the World. Your leadership skills, your ambition, your vision, your creativity, and your ability to share with others are amazing. Thank you so much for all you do in Tirana and Marikaj. I can't limit it just to the Hope Center, or to secretarial duties alone, because your talents touch many areas connected with the orphanages, local school system, the new church, the Bible classes to the kids, and the administrative duties. Your planning and organization for mission teams from America and other countries are such a blessing. It's a blessing to know the work you do to keep things running so smoothly at the Hope Center.

Thank you for your service, and thanks again for the part you have had in my book. I love you, GIG (girlfriend in God).

Thank you also to Anila Bushi Horner for your "Love Story" in my book. Thank you for making it a part of the book that most all girls will read first. We are grateful to God for allowing us to introduce you and Thad. We are thankful for your father-in-law, Dr. Jerry Horner, who led my husband, Roger, to Christ when they were both in their teens. God has a great way of putting people together and then bringing some wonderful miracles to pass in their lives in the future years. We feel this way about you, Anila. God bless you and Thad in your life together, and thanks again for sharing it with us in the *Albanian Attachment*.

And what could we have done without our sweet "grandfather image" employee for so long, Nikolin. We were so blessed to have you for the eighteen years before your retirement in your mid-seventies. Thanks, Nikolin, for adding to my book. Thanks for all the wonderful years we have enjoyed having you as a staff member. We love you and Nirvana and will always consider you as family of Hope for the World.

Cindy, my sweet daughter and office partner. I truly am at a loss for words as to how to properly thank you for taking time to write a piece for my book. I love you more than words can say and enjoy every minute spent with you in our work in the office, our out shopping, eating lunch, telling funny stories, doing music together and Bible studies, or anything else that we do together. You are the beat of my heart in so many ways. We talk over each other at the same time because we think alike. We have the same feelings and convictions on most everything. Thanks so much for being so much help to me daily, in the office and with family things. I love you and thank God for you every day, Cindy.

To Buddy and Kerri, what can I say? How special it is to have you also giving your lives 100 percent to missions of Hope for the

World. These past years you have taken on a huge burden for missions. Thank you for all of your encouragement and for your hard work. Thanks for the blessing you have been to all of us who direct the work of Hope for the World not only in Albania but also in Ethiopia, Honduras, India, the Philippines, Romania, and Ukraine. We pray for you as you try to bring these ministries to the forefront so churches and individuals can partner with us. You are truly a bright spot in our lives, not just in the mission endeavors. As our children, you bless us beyond measure. We are always thrilled by the music and songs that you write. Also with the addition of your two girls, our granddaughters, Victoria and Olivia, we are even more blessed. Thanks for loving Albania so much and for seeing to it that all of your family has visited there too so they can also feel that *Albanian Attachment.*

Last, but by no means least, to my life partner, the love of my life, *Roger*, I want to thank you so much for being my inspiration to put this book together. I appreciate the unselfishness you have displayed because of the many hours it has taken me to work; many hours and late hours, taking time we could have had together. You never complained one time. You added so much to my memories, and then your own thoughts and stories have been such a great addition to this book. You have gone through some really tough times during these years I have been writing. We have faced things we never ever thought we would face together. You have been true to your faith, true to me, and true to the family through everything. I love you more than I can ever put in words. I hope that through this book, many people will get to see the man that God called back in 1969 to begin a life of full-time Christian service. I hope and pray that your life's testimony will be a witness to many that no matter what age you are when God calls you, the only answer is *"yes."* You have truly been *the making of a wonderful life* for me, my honey.

Prologue

A History of Christianity in Albania

As I have been putting this book together, I have sought some assistance from Perparim Demcellari, our Albanian president of Hope for the World in Albania. With Perparim's help, rather than go to the encyclopedias and copy verbatim historical facts about Albania (which you can access and read at any time), I chose to share the history of Christianity in Albania. This is monumental, not only to Albania as a country but also to us as Bible-believing Christians. These next paragraphs were sent to me by Perparim, and I want to include them because they are of remarkable interest to believers of the Christian faith as well as affirming historical proof of the authenticity of the scriptures. It also tells us what an ancient country Albania is, which is another reason I love that country so much. Albania and Israel are truly the favorite places for me and my family to visit. I feel like I am truly in "God's country" when I am there.

According to Perparim, "Christianity spread in the territories inhabited by Albanians since the beginning of the first century". Several researchers believe that the apostle Paul, on his missionary journeys, evangelized these territories. In 56 AD, on Paul's third missionary journey, the Bible states that he was present in the territory of Illyria and Epirus (part of the Illyria territory). As to the actual territories in which he ministered, researchers believe that the apostle Paul preached and taught in Durres, Tirana, and Lezha. In his letter written to the Romans in 59 AD, Paul said: "So, from Jerusalem all the way around to Illyricum, I have fully proclaimed the gospel of Christ." Illyricum and Illyria are the ancient names for Albania. Even today, many people in Albania have names derived from that ancient name of their land. There are men named "Ilir" and women named "Liri." We personally know many people with these names.

The Italian researcher, Daniel Faloti, in his book *Ilirikum*, wrote that the church of Durres was founded by the apostle Paul. The bishop of this church in 58 AD having been Caesar was also known by the name Apollon. This bishop is mentioned in the apostle Paul's letter in Philippians 4:22.

The bishop of the church of Durres was sent to Rome at the same time Paul was in jail there. In the year 59 AD, in Durres, there were seventy in the Christian family. This is all information by researcher Daniel Faloti.

After Paul served his imprisonment in the jail at Rome, he returned back to Durres. Here he was awaiting Timothy, but since Timothy didn't arrive on time, he took with him the bishop of Durres, Apollon (Caesar), and they went together to the city of Nikopolis which was the Albanian city of Epir, where he met with Titus. Paul returned to Durres, and from there, he sent Titus to spread the gospel to Dalmatia (see 2 Timothy 4:10). There are many opinions that Paul wrote the letter to the Hebrews and that he wrote chapters 12 and 13 from Durres. Of course, we know that there has not been any real proof of who the writer of the letter to Hebrews was, but many theologians believe it was Paul.

The journeys of Paul to the actual territories of Albania have left signs through several toponyms (names derived from a topographical feature) and legends as well. For instance, in the capital city Tirana, there is a big area that includes fourteen villages named "Shen Paul," and historical studies say that Paul had stayed there. In Durres, there is also a small peninsula named "Kepi I Paulit."

In the city of Mirdite, there's a village named Shen Paul, and a rock is there that is named "Guri I prere I Shen Paulit." Legend has it that Paul broke the rock to open the road. In the south of Albania, there's a river named Paviloo (Paul). It is said that Paul traveled this river three times in the years 56, 62, and 63 AD. And also there was established a church which contains the name of the apostle Paul. In this church, it is said that Paul had performed baptisms.

It is also said that possibly Peter might have passed through and spread the gospel in Albania as well, since there are villages named "Shen Peter."

The third missionary journey of Paul to Albanian territory is included in the Italian maps printed in 1920–1945 and in the English maps printed in 1940–1950.

In the year 1965, the Second Council of the Vatican, in Rome, for some unknown reason, decided to ignore these maps that show the journeys of Paul.

Two American historians, Jacques, in his book entitled *Albanians*, and Roberts, in his book *World History*, also agree that the apostle Paul had been to, and had spread the gospel in, Albanian territory. Another historian from France, named Zhan Klod Foverid, in his book, *Albania History*, tells about the times of Paul in Albania.

I appreciate so much this information furnished by Perparim. Many thanks to him as he has been a great help to me in gathering these historical facts.

Along with the Apostle Paul, and other missionaries that have helped in the spreading of the gospel, there were also soldiers of Ilire (Albanian) origin who have helped in getting the gospel known in many places. There is also a very special missionary and personal friend of ours by the name of Gesina Secka Blaauw from Holland who has had a significant role in getting Hope for the World involved in the country of Albania soon after the iron curtain fell in that country. She also happens to be the missionary who sold us the property for our Hope Center for Teens in Marikaj, Albania. She has such a unique and interesting testimony about her beginnings with the Albanian people that I begged her to write her testimony about those days even before Albania opened up for missionaries to come there. She graciously agreed to do so, and I am inserting at the outset of this book what I am simply referring to as her testimony and entitling this chapter, "A Very Brave Missionary." I am so appreciative to her for sharing this with me so I could share it with you.

A Very Brave Missionary

By Gesina Blaauw

Brother Andrew

My name is Gesina Blaauw. I was born in Amsterdam, Netherlands, in 1952 and was born again spiritually in 1970 on Hershey's Poultry Farm in Troy, Ohio! The Lord immediately called me to serve him, and I took missionary training at the WEC Missionary Training College in Scotland from 1972 to 1974. From 1975 to 1991, I was a missionary in Sicily (Italy). My first visit to Albania was in 1981. It was such a shocking experience that my life would never be the same! Albania very much "became my life!"

How did I get involved with Albania? In 1975, I opened the Evangelical Bookshop in the capital of Sicily, Palermo. I was young and full of zeal, and the bookshop became a starting point for various other ministries. In December 1979, the field leader of our organization, CLC (Christian Literature Crusade), asked me to represent the entire Italian CLC ministry at the "Mission 80" Conference in Lausanne, Switzerland.

One of the main speakers there was *Brother Andrew*, who by then already was a friend of mine. We had gone to the same Missionary Training College in Scotland of the WEC. Actually, I had ended up there through reading his book, *God's Smuggler*.

This same book had touched *Enza*, a Sicilian lady who had come to know the Lord through our bookshop ministry. Now, she wanted to become a blessing to the ministry of Open Doors. Hearing that I was going to that conference and that *Brother Andrew* was going to speak there, she wrote him a letter and asked me to hand it to him.

There were twice as many young people at this conference as expected, and they could not all fit in the same meeting room. Therefore, every speaker now had to speak twice. I ended up in one meeting, with the Italians, while Brother Andrew that evening had been speaking to the English language group. Among all those seven thousand people, we "happened" to bump into each other on the steps of the main building. I asked him how his meeting had been, and his answer was, "It went very well. Thank you so much for your prayers!"

I told him I had a letter for him but it was not with me at that moment, and he asked me to bring it to his secretary at their Open Doors (OD) stand the next day.

His words about praying for him continued to go through my mind for the rest of that evening. I felt very guilty, because I really couldn't remember when I had last prayed for him! When I came to my bedroom, I knelt down before the Lord, and, repenting, I prayed: "Lord, please, from now on, make us a blessing to each other!"

The next day, I handed the letter to his secretary, Jan, and a very good friendship developed between us. When in Holland on furlough, I visited Jan and his family in what became my second home. It was very natural for me to invite them to Sicily for a holiday, never thinking that it would end up in ministry. While they were staying with me, the pastor of my village became ill and asked if my guest would speak during the meeting that Sunday. Jan shared testimonies of people from the suffering church in Eastern Europe, and people were touched by these testimonies. The word about this spread fast, and soon we received many invitations from other church groups. Jan then said to me that later on that year he would come back without his family and I could prepare meetings for him all over Sicily. We would also prepare an introductory edition of the Open Doors magazine in Italian. The meetings went so well that before we knew it, we had an Italian branch of OD and a full-time ministry involving several people.

Being so much involved, Jan suggested that I join a trip to Eastern Europe so I would personally know what it was all about instead of just from the testimonies of other people. Teams were leaving for Russia, but something in me said "Albania." I knew Albania was the hardest country in the world at that time. It even was officially atheistic! Also, in Sicily and southern Italy, there were many Arberesh villages. These were places where Albanian people had settled when the Ottomans conquered the Balkans in the fifteenth century. The Albanian hero, Skanderbeg, had helped the king of Naples and, as a reward, was offered these places for his people to settle in their flight from the Ottomans. Even today, these villages speak Albanian and have kept many Albanian traditions. I had friends from this minority group, so there was a link.

How to visit Albania was a different story and a matter for prayer. It seemed impossible! Traveling to other Eastern European countries, you could just go to the border and get a visa, but this was not the case for Albania. Then one day, I had to bring books to a church on the other side of Sicily. The meeting had already started when we arrived, but immediately, the speaker and the slides he was showing caught my attention. He had actually been in Albania and was showing slides about the country! After the meeting, we talked, and he explained to me that there was a communist organization which once a year organized a five-day group tour to Albania. And so it was that in September 1981, I entered Albania *with an Italian communist group!* With me was my Dutch bookshop colleague and friend, Marian. The Lord had shown us beforehand that we were to be very prudent and only to speak about him when he clearly told us to do so. We were to be very prayerful and alert to the leading of the Lord!

The first day in Albania was almost more than we could bear emotionally. Our hearts were longing to tell these people about the love of God. What we experienced on the streets was not just poverty, but what really hit us was the fear that radiated from their faces! We knew that probably there were microphones hidden in our room, so we went to the bathroom, turned on the tap to make noise, and then prayed together. *The Lord asked us right there if we were willing to lay down our life for these people, because for us, it was easy to talk and walk away, but they could be killed for those conversations. Both of us responded "yes."* From the next day on, the Lord gave us opportunities to speak on his behalf.

The Lord, through these conversations, in particular, had touched two people, and it was hard to leave them, we were walking out into liberty, but leaving them behind in their prison country! (One of these two we nicknamed Daniel, and he is still a very precious friend up until today.)

Back in Italy, for the first three or four days, we could only cry and pray and cry and pray. The Holy Spirit was burning God's burden and love for Albania on my heart.

More visits followed, and during the third trip, Daniel said to me: "You must come back to our country as often as you can, and you will receive inspiration."

During that same trip, I had also been able to lead another man to the Lord whose grandparents were born-again believers. I'll never forget his words: "When my grandparents die, there won't be anybody anymore to talk to me about God!" Immediately, I knew without any doubt that God would never allow that to happen. Every generation would receive an opportunity to hear the Gospel. I concluded, because of that, the time was near for God to open up Albania. Only he could do it. This conviction encouraged me to go out more into the open and ask believers everywhere in the world to pray for this in true intercession.

Full-Time for Albania: Breaking Down Barriers

Immediately after this trip, God showed me I was to go full-time for Albania to prepare the way and break down the barriers that existed between Albania and the free world. Before I knew it, there was an Italian missionary couple to take over the bookshop, and I was out giving my time fully to Albania. I already had begun to study the language after my first trip. Now I started translating articles of their own literature and pointing them to the influence of the Gospel on their society. I founded the Eagle's Club—the eagle being the symbol of Albania. But for me, it also means the Lord with his promise to carry me to the other side on the eagle's wings (Exodus) The Eagle's Club magazine came out in English, Dutch, and Italian and went to believers to stimulate them to pray. Copies also were sent to Albanian institutions and embassies as a testimony. It all came from their own literature and encyclopedias, so they couldn't oppose it.

Later on, after my prison experience which is described below, I moved to the Arberesh village of Piana degli Albanesi (Plain of the Albanians) and started an Albanian gift shop there, the Shqip Shop. Of course, the gift items had to be bought by us in Albania. By then, I also had a contract with the Albanian State Tourist Office, Albturist, and brought believers from various countries on tourist trips to Albania, where we would travel through the country and secretly pray for every place on which we stepped.

Once, we were refused to be given a visa because Albania had diplomatic problems with Italy about a family that had taken refuge in the Italian embassy. Instead of travelling inside of Albania, I took a small group of people to travel by car all around the borders of Albania, through Greece and what was then Yugoslavia. We tried to stay as close to Albania as we could, to pray, but also while travelling, we met many ethnic Albanians in those areas. They were also persecuted but for ethnic reasons. The Serbs hated Albanians, and also in Northern Greece, they were not allowed to speak their own language. We made many contacts but had no literature with us because we had counted on going into Albania. We promised each other, and the Lord, we would never travel to those places again without Biblical literature. In Pristina, Kosovo, a priest gave us some children's Bibles in Albanian and also New Testaments. In Yugoslavia, those things were legal, and they were even printed there.

One month later, I had to take another group into Albania. A week before that trip, I was to spend some days in Scotland for a Lydia Conference, where women from all over the world prayed for specific countries. I was to represent Albania there. I decided to bring my car over to Yugoslavia, have some days of rest, post some literature to people we had met a month earlier, and take a flight from Dubrovnik to Northern Europe. My car would then be waiting there so I could pick up the Dutch group after I came back to Yugoslavia and get into Albania as usual.

The Bread of Tears

The day before I left Sicily, the Lord had touched me through Psalm 80:5, "Thou hast fed them with the bread of tears." This Psalm was about the suffering of Israel, but to me, it spoke about the suffering of the Albanians.

It was the first time I travelled all alone to Yugoslavia. When I drove off the ferry, the police control seemed more intensive than usual. They continued to search my car, and I was losing a lot of time. Getting bored, I started to go through my correspondence. This drew their attention, and they also started to go through my correspondence. It seemed they were looking for an excuse to arrest me, and they found one! In my bag was a copy of a newsletter, where I reported about our last trip around the borders of Albania. In it was one sentence that they interpreted politically: "I have just come back from a trip, this time not inside of Albania, but still on Albanian territory." I had meant this in the ethnic sense, a people speaking Albanian and sharing the same Albanian culture and history, but now they accused me of being a spy for Albania!

They arrested me and interrogated me for many hours, but the Lord filled me with his peace that is above all understanding and even filled me with joy! I knew it would be impossible to convey these feelings to others. The questions they asked me gave me an opportunity to witness to them during most of the interrogation, and, because it was an official occasion, every word was written down! Toward the time the evening shift came to take over, they handcuffed me and then asked: "How do you feel?"

"What do you mean?" I asked.

"Well, aren't you angry? Aren't you afraid?"

"No, I want to learn."

"What do you want to learn?"

"I want to learn more from my Lord!" It was true, and I was full of joy and peace.

They could see that and exclaimed: "We have never met anybody like you before!"

They then handcuffed me to a desk in another office. After some hours, the men on the next shift, *Stephen and Sali*, said that they were sorry but now they had to bring me downstairs. These two had been very nice to me, bringing me food and drinks. Also, I had been able to tell Stephen that his name is in the Bible.

I would not be able to take anything with me, so I took out my contact lenses and went without them. Down the stairs, a terrible odor filled the place. They opened a cell door and closed it behind me. No light. Only darkness and a horrible stench filled the place. I felt my way toward a corner where a wooden plank offered a place to lie down. Because it had been a tiring day, I fell asleep.

When I woke up, I thought they would just let me go free, but I was to go through one of the deepest valleys of my life. I heard the footsteps of the guard coming downstairs and expected to be taken out by him. He opened the little spy hole in the metal door and made me understand I was to come near. It was dark in the cell, and I had forgotten there was a step somewhere near the entrance. I fell down as he opened the door. It was humiliating. When I got up, he put a piece of bread in my one hand and a piece of salami in my other hand and closed the door as well as the spy hole. It was utter darkness again!

It now dawned on me that I was nothing any more, not even a number. I was totally abandoned to the mercy of my enemies. Nobody in the whole world knew where I was or what had happened to me. I had disappeared from the scene. Humanly speaking, I was totally helpless! I made my way to the plank again and sat down to eat. How could I even eat? I needed one hand free to break the bread and tear off a piece of the salami, but where could I put anything? The stench was unbearable, and I couldn't see if there was any clean spot around me. As I sat there with the bread in my one hand and the salami in the other, the whole situation crashed in on me. Tears started to drop from my eyes and fell on the bread. Now the Lord reminded me of the *bread of tears*. The Lord Jesus himself had become a "bread of tears" for us, and also the body of Christ, his church, throughout the centuries had been a "bread of tears." Now I had become part of this bread of suffering, kneaded into the same dough. No longer was I an outsider praying for the suffering body of Christ, but I had become an insider. I experienced it now as *a baptism of suffering*, and I gained new strength and *authority for intercession* on behalf of the suffering church. I gained *new intimacy with the Lord Jesus!* That day became a day of intercession. I prayed for every communist country I could think of. I was fighting the spiritual fight effectively! He turned one of my lowest moments into one of the highest!

On the third day, they brought me to court, and the judge officially gave me another thirty days in prison. Then the secret police interrogated me again and said they had the last word and that I would die in prison. They transferred me to a real prison in Spuz, near Titograd (nowadays called Podgorica). I had asked the judge if I could contact the embassy and my mother, and he had said yes, but his words and the law were not respected. I wrote, but my letters were held back. I realized this when no answers came.

The first moments in zatvor (prison) Spuz impressed me. When the guard brought me into the women's quarters, everybody jumped up on their feet and stood still. That was the rule of respect! I made up my mind right away that I would not allow myself to have self-pity but would honor the Lord and learn from him and grow closer to him.

They had taken everything away from me, so I had no watch, no Bible, nothing, apart from a book that I had accidently left in a bag. The women around me didn't know the Lord, and we had nothing in common. I didn't know their language either, but one of them knew some words in German and another knew some words in Albanian. The woman guard in charge of us also wanted to communicate, and she took a booklet along of "how to speak in Serbo-Croatian" with everyday sentences in English and Serbo-Croatian. This was helpful to try and have some conversation. Once, I pointed to the sentence: "Do you know where is…?" and pointed to heaven.

She answered, "No, I don't know."

I then said, "What do you call this?" pointing to the wall.

"Mur."

"You here, God there, wall between. Wall sin, need door. Jesus door. Door not automatic!"

It would take many pages to write about many special moments, situations, and lessons I learned during prison time. The Lord was very close to me. During the evenings, knowing that for quite a long time no guard would enter our room, I would climb on a chair, and from there, on the windowsill, hold onto the bars that were there to prevent us from escaping. In that position, I could look over the outside prison wall and see the stars. The bright polar star was right in front of me, and I would fix my eyes on it, and worship Jesus, the morning star. I would sing out loud because the ladies around me were worshipping Satan in their magic actions, reading the future in their cigarette stumps, or reading cards. By then, they had understood the point, and when they pulled out their cards, they would look at me and say: "Gesina, Satan!" Just standing there singing, praising, and praying for them always made them quiet, and if I didn't do it, they would ask me to sing. They really quarreled when I did not sing.

Sometimes, they provoked me to see my reactions, like Zorga, who looked at me and then picked up Anna's cup of tea and spat in it while Anna walked over to the window to watch the cat with her kittens that were in the garden. Zorga and Anna hated each other. I quietly took the cup and replaced it with a fresh cup of tea. Anna never knew what had happened.

During my first days in zatvor Spuz, my mind was set on how to be able to escape because they had threatened that I would be there the rest of my life and I would die in prison. That's why I knew it was not my imagination when the Lord spoke very clearly these words to me: "I don't want you to be anxious. I will send you two angels, and you will know exactly what to do!"

These words totally broke through my own thoughts. I decided to believe and act according to these words and just trust the Lord. If the angels would be heavenly angels or human messengers, I didn't know, but the Lord would somehow intercede in my situation.

Four weeks later, a guard told me, "Two men were asking for you this afternoon."

I rejoiced. The angels had come! Nothing happened the next day, and I prayed that the Lord would make these people stay and not go away. I didn't know that nobody in the world knew where I was. *Maybe they have come to this area on business and want to visit me*, I thought. I prayed that they would be there at the moment I would maybe be transferred to another prison, so that I would be able to shout out to them what happened and they could do something about it. Another day went by, and nobody turned up. When that same guard was on duty again, I asked him what these men looked like. When he described them, I had an impression that maybe I knew one of them. The guard had sent them to the high court to obtain permission for them to visit me. Saturday came, and the lady guard was on duty. She called me out and told me to pack my things and come to her office. Were they going to transfer me before my visitors could speak with me? Again, I prayed that they would be there. Once in her office, she said that I was free to go. I asked for a taxi, but that was not allowed, she said. I insisted because of my disability and the many suitcases that had been kept at the police station and had to come back with me. She had to ask the director. When coming back she exclaimed, "Your friends really love you!" I looked amazed, and she continued, "If it wasn't for them, you would not be free. They are here, go outside!"

As soon as I stepped through the door, a man I didn't know came and embraced me whispering at my ear, "Pretend that you know me and that you don't know the other person in the car." The man at the wheel was a precious friend of mine, but I played the game and kept my distance. There was another person in the car, apparently to spy on them. Once we had dropped him in Titograd (Podgorica), we stopped in a quiet place to talk, thanked the Lord, and asked for his directions because we were not out of danger yet.

My car and passport were still in the town of Bar, where I was arrested, at the police station. That is where the secret police had been tough on me and had threatened me and said that they had the last word. We asked the Lord whether we had to go there or better not and go to Belgrade to the Dutch embassy to ask for their protection and a travel document. All three of us felt we had to go to Bar. It was the end of the summer season. No rain had fallen for several months, but now, just as we entered the town, it started pouring rain. This covered us from sight and also it made people stay indoors. When we approached the police station, we decided that one of the men would accompany me and the other one would stay at a safe distance with the car, so that if we didn't come back within a certain time, he could warn the embassy. Only one person manned the police station when we came, and, to my great joy, it was Stephen! I was now able to thank him for his kindness, which had meant a lot to me. He gave back my passport and other belongings, including the New Testaments and Gospels that had been with me, and handed me the car keys. No stamp in my passport. Everything was like normal and like nothing had happened.

The men decided that one of them would drive my car. The next evening, we were to cross the border between Yugoslavia and Austria. As we approached the border, we decided that I would drive my car on my own and the others would follow at a safe distance so that if anything happened to me, they could warn the embassy. These were communist days, and crossing the border of an Eastern European country took time and bureaucracy. I still was in third gear when a man without a cap, with long blond hair, stepped out on the road in front of me and signaled that I had to drive on. In third gear, without slowing down, I drove out of Yugoslavia and into the free world. Nobody had checked on me! This must have been an angel from heaven! When I looked behind me, the men had been stopped and were subjected to all the normal border checks.

These two men both were involved in Brother Andrew's mission. Open Doors had been standing close with my mother and offered her all the encouragement they could. (Like if she needed to identify my dead body somewhere, they would accompany her!) When after more than three weeks, the international police had not been able to find me, these two brothers felt they should go personally and search for me. Open Doors organized around-the-clock prayer for ten days, and they were to come back with my body or with news about me.

Their trip was dangerous, so they needed prayer, but nobody was supposed to know their names. Open Doors communicated to these prayer warriors that they had to pray for "the two angels." They had no idea what the Lord had told me!

Interrogated in Albania

Less than one month later, I was on my way to Albania again to accompany the group that was planned for September. While I was in prison in Yugoslavia, the August group had continued their journey in Albania without me. Albania too knew that something had happened to me. Actually, I believe that the same person, who had warned the Yugoslav authorities against me, had also informed the Albanian authorities. Right from the beginning, we were always followed by an extra vehicle and extra agents in our bus. ("The men with the brown shoes!") About three days before the end of this trip, the agency representative told me that the group was going on their trip without me that day because there would be an interview with me. In the past, I had given interviews for Radio Tirana so that's what I expected this time also, but I soon understood that this time it was the Albanian secret police that wanted to hear me out!

Three officers and an interpreter (one of the tour guides from another group) took me along in the elevator to the top floor of the highest building of Tirana at that time, the Hotel Tirana. These men were not all unknown to me. I had been praying for a man whom I had seen a few times at the Albanian embassy in Rome. He looked like the most miserable person in the world. I had never seen such an unhappy and unhealthy-looking person. He was a very high-level secret service person. Now he was right here in the room for the interrogations! For me, this was an answer to prayer. Four out of the six hours of interrogation, I was able to share the Gospel with them. Again, I experienced perfect peace and joy. The Lord was right there. There were three sessions of two hours each. One of the questions during the first session was: "What do you think of our system?"

I told them I appreciated their health system and their educational system, but of course this was not what they meant.

They then changed the question into, "What do you think of our doctrine?"

Here I could say that Marx and Lenin started change from the outside but Jesus from the inside. I also explained that I hated religion but loved Jesus, and they wanted to know the difference.

"How can you believe in what you cannot see?"

My answer: "Do you love your wife?"

"Of course, I do!"

"But I cannot see that!" The window was open, and the wind was blowing and moving the curtain. That was another illustration: "You cannot see God, but you can see what he is doing!"

During one of these intervals, they asked if I wanted to drink something, but I didn't want to go to the café on my own. Then they sent the interpreter, Artan, along with me. I knew the things he heard had touched him. I asked him if it had been difficult for him to interpret these conversations, and he answered that the language was not difficult but the concepts were new to him. The Lord touched Artan, and some months later, he became a refugee.

When we were all in the elevator again to start the third session, one of the officers asked me, "Are we going to heaven or to hell?" These men had never had an opportunity to hear about God, and I was very happy to have this opportunity to share with them now!

The third session was not so nice. Things became serious now. They asked me about a refugee that I had helped. We had nicknamed him *Jonah* because he had spent much time in the water before being picked up by a Greek ferryboat. I had met him in a refugee camp in Italy. He was always very sad and thinking about his family that he had left behind. I kept telling him that God would one day reunite them again, but he thought that would never happen. He also was very hungry for the things of God. He became involved in translating the Psalms into Albanian, and later on, he did the proofreading and corrections on the New Testament that an English linguistic missionary had translated who had never been in Albania. Being friends with somebody who had illegally left the country automatically made me their enemy. They told me to tell him he would never see his country alive any more. They also said that I could no longer come into Albania. They gave me a stern warning to never meet refugees again. I now was blacklisted!

The next day, when our group had a coffee stop on our way to the north, another tour bus stopped alongside ours. To my surprise, one of the people on the bus was the interpreter of the day before, Artan. He wanted to encourage me and told me not to worry. With him was his colleague and best friend, Andrea Opari. Both escaped the country some months later, and we were able to help and employ them in Holland in a translation agency we set up for this purpose. They worked on the translation of the *Children's Bible* by Anne DeVries, which we would need when the doors of Albania opened up some years later. Andrew's escape and trip to Holland is another interesting story, which would take several extra pages!

Persona Non Grata

Blacklisted by the Albanians, but Not by the Lord!

Now I was in a situation where I would not be able to travel to Albania again. This was very discouraging, but the Lord kept saying that he had called me to be involved with Albania, and one day, I would live there and be involved in its rebuilding. I needed to walk by faith! For me, that meant to continue learning the language and to continue with the Eagle's Club. I moved to the Arberesh village of Piana degli Albanesi. The Lord started bringing people together from all over the world that had a burden for Albania. Each one had kept it a secret because it was dangerous and there were many spies around. Ever since my third trip into the country, I had started to proclaim that Albania would soon be free. Now, many churches invited me, and I shared about Albania not only in my home country of Holland but also in Britain, Norway, the United States, Germany, Switzerland, and even in Nigeria (Africa).

The Lord was working out his plan and raised up an army of prayer warriors. One meeting in Norway, humanly speaking, would have been unimpressive with only about twelve people present, but the Lord doesn't look at numbers. An elderly man started crying and came to me afterward, saying he had a print shop and had the impression the Lord wanted him to print the New Testament in Albanian if we could provide him with the text. I told him about the translation that was being proofread by Jonah. I also told him that for the moment, the country was still closed, but it would open soon and we had to have spiritual food ready to hand out when that moment came! One or two years later, they called me and told me they had printed seventy thousand copies and asked if I could now help bring them in. We needed to wait for the Lord's moment!

It was during this time of being blacklisted by Albania that many interesting people came my way, Albanians as well as people from all over the world with a heart for Albania. One of those was Jimmy Franks. He lived in Germany at that time and was in touch with Open Doors.

Just after I moved to the Arberesh village, it celebrated its five hundred years of existence, and many activities had been organized for this occasion. That year, we had an Albanian dance group visiting us along with a linguistic congress. I was invited to every occasion because by now, they considered me an "Albanologian." There were always people with those groups to spy on them but still, the Lord gave good contacts and many conversations. During the linguistic congress, I had filmed some of the speakers. From the University of Tirana, there was the famous professor, Andrea Kostallari, together with his assistant, Professor Agim Hiddi. It really clicked between Agim and me, and I asked him if he wanted to see the video of him speaking. He said yes, and we made use of the lunch break to go to my apartment. I am a lover of books, and as soon as he walked in, Agim saw the Albanian books in my library. His eyes immediately fell on the New Testament portion in Albanian that had just been printed. He asked permission to read it and said the language was beautiful. When walking around the house, he saw a picture of my friend in Niger, a Sicilian missionary named Leonardo Navarra. Leonardo had adopted more than forty children, and they were all together in this picture. This story touched Agim's heart. Some years later, when Albania opened up, Agim immediately became involved with us. He, along with his wife, proofread and edited the Old Testament. Both of them became believers during this process! They hosted many missionary visitors in their home in Tirana from May 1991 when the doors opened for us till they immigrated to the United States. Agim also became secretary of the newly established Albanian Evangelical Alliance (VUSH).

Jonah's Story Continued

Lee Young had been travelling all over Europe for half a year, trying to find somebody who would be able to do the programs of "Words of Hope" in Albanian. When he asked me if I knew a person who could do this, my thoughts went to Jonah. It was an answer to a prayer. Jonah had received his papers for the United States shortly after my interrogations in Albania and just in time to escape the threats of the person who had also betrayed me. The Lord was very clearly in charge of all of these details and in every move we made in those days. Jonah became the translator and broadcaster for Words of Hope for several years and, after that, up until the present time, worked for the Albanian branch of Voice of America.

When the Berlin Wall came down, it also had its effect on Albania little by little. The real turning point came when a truck full of people drove right through the wall of the Italian embassy and all asked for asylum in Italy. Thousands of people followed their example, and they stormed and invaded every western embassy in Tirana. The whole world became involved, and emergency measures were taken for various countries to accept these refugees. Refugee camps were arranged in Italy where many escaped to on boats. Refugees crowded every ship they could find, fighting their way to get on board. Many people, especially infants, drowned and died during these attempts. For my part, I got in touch with the missions that had been printing materials in the Albanian language, and we were able to send thousands of copies to churches and individuals that became involved in working with these refugees.

I called Jonah in America and told him that if his family was among them, they could live with me till their papers were ready.

"That can never happen," he said. But three days later, I was informed that they were all there! Among the refugees were his wife, his two children, and two of his brothers as well as their cousin and husband. They were in a refugee camp in Bari, Italy. From there, refugees were spread out to other places.

With the coordinating authorities of Piana degli Albanesi, I was able to arrange that Jonah's family would stay in my house. I picked them up when the refugee bus arrived. A new season of ministry began, working with the refugees.

Jonah had always been telling me about his little girl, Romina, who was five years old when he left the country. He also had a baby boy but did not realize this boy was disabled. Jonah's little son, Stephen, was the first Albanian child I met with a disability.

As soon as we were in my house, Romina asked me, "Do I look like my father?"

It still touches my heart to think of the love between them and how the Lord brought them back together. We called Jonah in the United States. How wonderful to see them get reconnected!

I started English lessons for refugees, and a small group met at my house every day for a few hours. During these lessons, I was able to tell them about the Lord Jesus, and we had several baptisms in the months that followed. The refugees had spread out to other Arberesh villages and towns around Palermo. Visiting them and the churches that worked with them also became part of the program. Sometimes, it meant travelling to Rome with refugees to help them with their refugee documents, interviews, etc.

Meanwhile, Daniel, who had remained a good friend ever since the first trip in 1981, had asked me to help his younger brother, Arben, who had a problem with his eyes and was almost blind. If I could find a specialist willing to operate on him, maybe the authorities would grant a visa for him and also his family members to accompany him. My mother's eye specialist looked at the info I provided and referred me to the best professor in Holland, Dr. Worst. He agreed to do the surgery and issued a written invitation for Arben to come to Holland. In March 1991, I left the refugees behind in my home in Sicily and drove to Bari to pick up Daniel's brothers and sister from the ferry. We drove straight on to Holland to my mother's home where we stayed during Arben's months of surgery and recovery.

Albania wanted to become part of the United Nations and were told that they needed to respect international human rights, one of which was freedom of religion. Albania agreed to do so. This promise needed to be tested of course. Also, Albania opened a new embassy in Scandinavia, and the people who had printed the New Testament went to the embassy requesting a visa and permission to bring in medicines, clothes, and New Testaments. The permission was granted, the visas were given, and they phoned me to tell me to send them my passport as well. A few days later, the miracle was done; my passport came back with a visa! I was no longer on the "blacklist." The last time I had been in Albania was four years earlier at which time I had been interrogated by the secret police for six hours. My prayer had been that the Lord would place me on the opposite list one day, and he did!

The Breakthrough: First Week of May 1991

The day after I received my passport with the visa, we loaded my car, called Daniel, and arranged for me to stay in his home. His father waited for me at the border. So now, I had one Albanian refugee family staying in my home in Sicily, one Albanian family staying with my mother in Holland, and me staying in the home of their parents in Albania!

The Scandinavian-German team had asked me to lead the conversations with the authorities because I knew the culture and language. They had arrived one day before I did and were staying in the Tirana Hotel (where I had been interrogated three and a half years earlier!). I met them the morning after my arrival. They already had taken an interpreter and arranged for some official meetings to take place with government officials.

The interpreter, Joseph, opened his heart to the Lord right from the beginning. We had meetings with, among others, the Minister of Culture, Sports and Education, the Minister of Health, and the Head of the Advisors of the Prime Minister. We also had some literature with us to give to each one of them: the New Testament and a book written in the beginning of the nineteenth century by the Albanian Evangelical Christian, Gjerasim Qiriazi. To our great surprise, each one of these high government officials told us that the country really needed this and that their spiritual need was even greater than the material need! We could share the Gospel with them, talking about forgiveness in Christ and new life in Christ.

I will never forget the look on the face of Thoma Qiriasi, the head of the Advisors of the Prime Minister. He looked so lost but also was so open! During our second visit to him, we asked if we could receive permission to start a full-time activity to encourage the people of Albania materially as well as spiritually.

"Why not?" Thoma answered.

"Then we need offices and warehouses for relief supplies," we told him.

"We will supply you with all of these!" was his answer.

We then stated, "Another thing is that we would like for the entire population to hear this message of forgiveness that we have shared with you, so that in Albania, there won't be a bloodbath like we saw in Romania."

He replied, "Nothing against that."

We asked, "Can we use the football stadium for that purpose?"

He answered, "Why not?"

We asked, "Then, when can we do this?"

He stated, "The football season finishes at the end of June, so the stadium will be free in July. You can do it the first week of July!" Thoma then added, "But if you are going to organize all of these activities and you have to invite many foreigners into this country, we need somebody to stand between the foreigners and our government. Can you be that person?"

And so the Lord answered my prayer to get me off the "blacklist" and on the opposite list. Now I was authorized to invite people in and get visas for them. The door was now wide open! These were historic moments. The situation in the country was reversed at that moment, and the light of God was officially allowed to come in and invade the darkness.

The team asked me to stay behind in Albania to organize everything on the spot while they gathered together as many missionary organizations as possible to put together a joint effort to reach out to Albania on a permanent basis. We also wanted to encourage them spiritually as well as materially, as we had promised the government we would do. A meeting was planned for the end of May in Lidkoping, Sweden. I was to make pictures of all the things the Albanian government had promised and which had to materialize before this meeting took place. It would convince everybody that Albania was open and that the facilities were ready for the work to begin there.

The team left, and there I stood in Hotel Tirana, overwhelmed and all alone, facing an enormous task for which we had prayed for so many years! I asked the Lord to do another miracle and to send me at least one person that could help me and be a prayer partner. After this prayer, I started to leave the hotel and was almost outside when I heard a woman's voice calling my name. Could this be possible? Yes, there was Nashua, a Brazilian missionary who had been serving the Lord in Kosovo, waiting for Albania to open. Somehow, she had heard that I was there. We had met in the past in Kosovo. She had obtained a visa for Albania but had to leave the country now. She had been praying for the Lord to do a miracle and provide her with another visa! Here, we were joined together by the Lord. Nashua obtained her visa, and I obtained my first coworker. Together, we went for it! For the stadium event, we would need as many Albanian-speaking missionaries as we could find, and there were not many available. Nashua knew all of those who were waiting in Kosovo for the doors to open. We contacted all of them and invited them for the stadium event in July. We prepared their visa applications and also started contacting many other people that had been praying and waiting for this moment.

The Albanian government provided us with offices and warehouses. We obtained permission to print *The Father Heart of God* by Floyd McClung, a book that Jonah's younger brother had translated while staying in my home in Sicily. We brought it to an Albanian company to print. Victory on every level!

We had meetings with the director of the stadium who said, "Whenever we use the stadium for a special event, we have banners made to put out in the streets. You must make banners!"

When praying and asking the Lord what would be effective, he reminded me of the general mind-set of the people we had met in the streets during these days. Many would say, "God has forsaken us because we have turned our back to him!" The opposite was true of course. He had opened the doors in a miraculous way because he loved the people of Albania and because people from all over the world had been interceding for them in prayer throughout the years. God loved them, and he loved Albania. To break through this mind-set that said that God had forsaken them, we had the banners made with the proclamation: "God Loves Albania!" The banners were hung up by the state enterprise. This time, no communist banners! Only banners proclaiming that God loves Albania! They placed these banners not only near and at the stadium but also in every entry road to the city as well as on the main squares of Tirana. Very quickly, the word spread throughout the country that in Tirana, people were talking about God. People came walking from faraway places just to meet with us.

Carrying pictures of the warehouses and the stadium, I went to Sweden for the meeting at the end of May. Mission leaders from many organizations had come, and we rejoiced together while making plans on how to proceed. It was important to present ourselves as a cohesive unit and not as many separate denominational groups. We needed each other to fulfill the task of encouraging the Albanian people spiritually as well as materially. We needed each other for the stadium event and for building up Albania. We decided to create a common platform under the name "Albanian Encouragement Project." This name was nonthreatening because it avoided the word "mission." We formed two groups within this platform, one to coordinate the spiritual start at the stadium and one to coordinate the relief work.

The Albanian government gave us the premises of the Blind Institute to use during the stadium event. We used it to host the teams and as our offices. We also parked the buses there that were brought by the Norwegians. They would load these buses full of relief supplies, and I could write several pages about adventurous events as people were chasing us because they wanted the boxes they could see through the bus windows. It really was a Wild West story but in Albania. It was normal for us to literally be at gunpoint or to have stones thrown at us. One man, who had put a pistol to my head, later became a friend. He attended every meeting at the stadium, and later we planned a distribution of relief supplies at the city quarters where he lived (and "ruled!")

The stadium event during the first week of July 1991 was very significant. The meetings were at night because daytime was too hot. Every evening, we announced that everybody who wanted to know more about God could come for Bible studies under the trees of Tirana, meeting near the steps of the university every morning. Many small groups would be gathered under the trees, in the parks, and in the squares. It reminded me of the time of Nehemiah and Ezra when they were teaching the entire population to fear the Lord. At the end of the stadium events, we announced baptisms at the artificial lake of Tirana. Again, this was an event never to be forgotten. I felt like I was watching John the Baptist. Every person who wanted to be baptized first had to give a personal testimony. Soldiers with guns were standing by because they were guarding the park. Some of them were so touched by these testimonies and God's word that they put their guns on the ground and also entered the water to be baptized. The same happened to a filmmaker of the official film studio, Kinostudio. He handed his camera to somebody else and was baptized.

From these meetings, the first church began. It immediately had about four hundred members, and the missionary in charge was totally overwhelmed, because in Kosovo, he only had a church of twenty! Right from the beginning, it was decided that, after a certain period, part of this group would become a second church under the care of another missionary. Soon, other churches were started in other cities of Albania.

I became very much a voice making known the needs of Albania all over the world. Communications went mainly by fax at that time. I used the fax machines of various ministries to send out appeals for help. One fax on August 9, 1991, included an invitation to Jimmy Franks. It was in Dutch, sent by me to an Open Doors secretary and then translated into English. One part went "(3) I would like to see Jimmy Franks involved with the humanitarian work. I only have his phone number and no fax. Could you please communicate to him everything that has happened? Tel. 0049-6187-22262." This was one of five points included in that fax.

Jimmy came quite soon, and I remember he brought an overhead projector for the church. He told me about people who had started projects for orphans in Romania and asked if he could involve them. He came back with other men of God, and we made a proposal to the Albanian government, starting off again at Thoma Qiriasi's office and forwarded by him to the Ministry of Health and Education. Many months of negotiations followed. It was complicated because we had to deal with both ministries, but the result was that Hope for the World began taking care of the orphanages in Albania, and they are still doing so today!

Their first missionaries stayed in my house until they found other accommodations. Also, I was able to link a Dutch charity with the Tirana orphanage, and they did some rebuilding projects, renewed the bathrooms, etc. Others provided food that we could deliver to the orphanage, and Hope for the World missionaries always were warm friends to have around. I loved it when they would invite me to their apartment at the orphanage for fellowship.

Now, it is the end of 2014, and we are handing over to Hope for the World the place in Marikaj that for many years was our headquarters where we rehabilitated young people with physical disabilities. I am so happy that the mission work continues and that this property is in Christian hands! We ourselves still have a piece of land adjacent to this property, and I look forward to us being able to be a blessing to each other in the future!

Author's Note

I thank my friend, Gesina, for this very interesting documentation of her early years in setting the stage for Hope for the World and other missionaries to be able to come into Albania and begin what has become a great work since that time. I will tell you more about Gesina's property that has become our Hope Center for Teens a little later on in this book. I will now begin my own writings and add in other testimonies as God brings them to my mind. I want to give all the glory and praise to our heavenly Father for these years that he has allowed us to be a part of the ongoing mission in the beautiful country of Albania, touching lives, changing hearts, and making a real difference, especially in the lives of the orphans as well as many others. To God be the glory!

I trust you will be blessed by what you find in these pages, and I would just ask that you breathe a prayer as you read that God will continue growing "his kingdom" in the hearts and lives of countless Albanians, for his glory. What an awesome day it will be when we gather around his throne and find a great congregation there from this beautiful country. It's gonna be worth it!

The years from 1994 until now have made a great impact on Roger and me and the lives of our children and grandchildren. We would not exchange one day, one night, and one mile walked, driven, or flown during this time. It's all been good because God is so good, all the time!

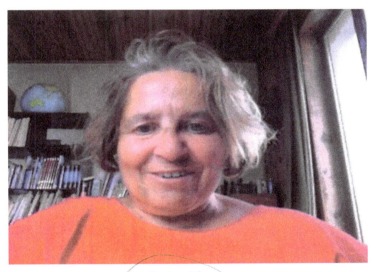

Gesina Blaauw
"A Very Brave Missionary"

Making of a Wonderful Life Albanian Attachment

Hope for the World: The Beginning

On November 9, 1989, when the Berlin Wall fell, Pastor Jimmy Franks and his wife, Janice, were sitting in their living room in Central Florida making plans to move to Europe to be missionaries. They were pastoring a church at that time and had been travelling back and forth to Europe for almost twenty years doing Bible conferences there. Gradually, their hearts' passion shifted toward sharing Christ with Europe in a more hands-on way. When the wall fell, Jimmy said that he felt like this was a sign from the Lord. "It was like it was torn down for us to go."

They moved to Germany in the summer of 1990. Soon after the Berlin Wall fell in 1989, the "Romanian Revolution" occurred. It was a violent revolution, but as a result, the door to Romania was opened.

Jimmy states, "We began to immediately travel back and forth from Germany to Romania holding crusades and sharing Christ's love in Romania. Previously, Romanians did not have much of any Christian witness or any Bible-teaching churches. There were thousands of villages of all different sizes where the Romanian people had seldom, or never, heard the story of Christ and the crowds coming to these crusades were spectacular. The response was incredible."

The country of Albania, under the dictatorship of Enver Hoxha, had actually listed itself with the United Nations as an atheistic country with absolutely no religions, and it remained so throughout Hoxha's regime, until the year 1991, when communism fell in Eastern Europe. At that time, Jimmy and Janice surrendered to be missionaries in Europe. Being burdened for people who never had access to the Bible before, and seeing the open door for the first time to share the message of Christ with those people, Jimmy founded the organization "Hope for the World." HFTW actually started in Romania with crusades and teaching Romanian pastors. Then, seeing the poverty and the need to care for orphaned children, the "Villages of Hope" were established to care for orphans in that country.

It was during that first year in Romania that Jimmy received a phone call from a lady named Gesina who was a missionary in Sicily to the Albanian refugees. It was amazing that God had providentially caused their paths to cross in Florida several years before while Jimmy was still pastoring a church. She had stayed in their home and asked them to put Albania on their prayer list. Albania was a country Jimmy didn't know much about. He wasn't even sure where it was located in Europe. He began to research Albania and found that four million people were indoctrinated to be totally atheistic, they had adopted communism, they outlawed any religion, and they had concentration camps for those who dared to practice a religion of any kind. Political dissidents were placed in these concentration camps under conditions so horrific that many died there.

When Brother Jimmy received this call from Gesina, she told him Albania had undergone a revolution, and she asked if he would consider coming to Albania and letting her introduce him to the country with the possibility of helping her bring the message of Christ to Albania.

Jimmy recalls, "With fear and trembling, I bought a ticket to Tirana, Albania. The airlines did not even know what paperwork I needed because tourism was not allowed in Albania. I flew into Tirana and was met by soldiers with AK-47s. They asked for my paperwork and, of course, I did not have what was needed, and I was escorted into the miniscule plane terminal, such as it was, and assured I would be put in jail or sent back on the next plane. Then Gesina, my guardian angel, came to my rescue with my paperwork and a visa.

"Gesina had arranged a place for me to stay that night with the former Minister of Health. The next day we had prayer with Gesina, two Campus Crusade missionaries, and one other Operation Mobilization missionary. We prayed for God to continue to open doors in Albania. From there, they took me to meet a cabinet member in the government of Albania. I will never forget that meeting, because he was very open to anything we wanted to do. I asked him to help us find a building in which to start a church. I remember I even had to explain to him what a church was. He was very kind but said it would be very hard to give us a building since people were coming out of the concentration camps and coming back into the cities from the mountains where they had fled, and there was very little room, if any, in the buildings they had to use for these people. We then discussed the orphanages where the children and babies lived and how deplorable the conditions were there.

"We walked through the baby orphanage in Tirana. The place had no heat. It was so cold you could see the freezing breath from the babies' little mouths and noses. They were in cribs wearing cloth diapers that hadn't been changed and had very little to eat besides some watery soup. It was a disturbing and emotional experience to know these babies would probably not live to grow up and one day leave these orphanages. They would most likely die from exposure and malnutrition. The government official then asked me to take over their orphanages, 'We will just give them to you, and you can take them over and help the children. If you do this, there is a chapel in the school-age orphanage in Tirana that is located right across the street from the American embassy. You can use that chapel to start a church.' We went and looked at the chapel and found it was fairly large and, unbelievably, in pretty good condition for that period of time in Albania.

"I sought counsel from a couple of pastors in the USA, and we agreed to provide for the orphanages in Tirana. We trusted God for the needed funds to support the renovations and the food needed to care for these children. At the same time, we planted our first church in Albania. It was like starting from scratch in a country that had not had the Gospel for nearly fifty years. None of these children knew a thing about Jesus Christ. His name had not been allowed to cross their lips in Albania under the communist dictatorship. Those who were caught trying to practice Christianity had been either killed or sent to labor camps as prisoners.

"Many of the kids from the school-age orphanage came to our church, and many of them came to know Christ. What a joy it was to teach them about Jesus and his virgin birth. It wasn't too long before these children from the orphanage put on their very first Christmas pageant in that chapel! Several government officials came to see this program, and since Albania was declared atheistic since 1947, they had never heard the true meaning of Christmas. Can you imagine how blessed we were to see the orphans making this first presentation of Christ to their government leaders?"

Jimmy and Janice moved back to the United States in order to raise the money needed to take care of these orphans.

Jimmy said, "We really didn't set out to take care of orphans, but when we saw the orphanages, we knew that God dropped them into our laps to help them. These children were literally the key to the door of the Gospel opening in Albania at that time. How could we expect to share Christ with the Albanian people if we did not first care for, feed, and clothe these poor children? This was where the dream and vision for Hope for the World was born, created by the need to have a ministry for these orphans, as well as all the other ministries that would gradually become a part of Hope for the World.

"In the beginning stages of Hope for the World, and because there was such an urgent need for help in Albania with the orphanages, volunteer workers were sought to go and give their time freely to the cause. Many of them were Christian people who were retirees and had their own source of income. There were no funds from Hope for the World to provide any salaries or expenses for them. They had to have a heart to help, and this they did willingly.

"Some American college students also gave their summers to go as missionaries and assist on projects of restoration to the Tirana orphanage. They would double their duties from labor on the building repairs to ministering to the complex needs of the orphan children in this government institution. Though the children were starving and cold, it was obvious that one of their biggest needs was for someone to love them. They were not receiving any love from the government employees. This group of volunteers was actually burning themselves out very quickly because of the heavy load of physical work as well as the emotional pull of the suffering children in this, the poorest country in Eastern Europe.

"They were a wonderful group of men and women who went way above and beyond their call of duty to touch the lives of about 170 children who were living in the Zyber Hallulli Orphanage in Tirana at the time, together with another large group of deaf children that was also seeking their help. The American embassy had been established in 1991 right across the street from the orphanage in Tirana. It gave us a sense of protection to have it close by, and in a few years, it actually proved itself to be a great source of protection to the children and our missionaries."

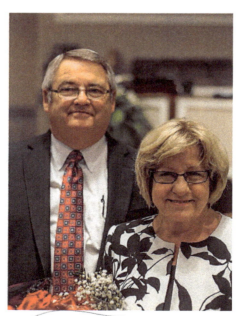

Jimmy and Janice Franks
Founders of Hope for the World Missions

Roger's Calling to Albania

In March of 1994, my good friend, Jimmy Franks, called me and asked me to accompany Marvin Lane, our mutual friend who was working in missions to Eastern Europe, to Albania. We were going there to look over the work that had been started recently under Hope for the World, a newly formed 501(c)3 nonprofit organization of which Jimmy Franks was the president. I had some time free and was interested in seeing the work that they were doing over there. Cherie and I had earlier been on a mission trip to Romania with Brother Jimmy and his wife, Janice, along with other missionaries connected with Hope for the World. We knew that doors were opening in these formerly communist dictatorships, and Hope for the World was one of the first American organizations to enter these countries with the Gospel since the iron curtain had fallen.

Our route to Albania was from America to Budapest, Hungary, and then on to Albania from Budapest. As it is in many airports in Europe and other countries, the airlines used a tram or bus to transfer passengers from the plane to the airport terminal once they had landed. I had been standing close to the door waiting to exit from one of these people movers when it stopped, and I started to get off with my briefcase in hand. The rush of the people trying to get off the bus pushed me out the door, and I went sprawling onto the pavement face-first, losing my grip on my briefcase. I tried to catch myself on my hands when I fell, and in so doing, I felt a terrible shock go up through my arms and elbows which completely knocked me out for a few seconds. My traveling companion and friend, Marvin Lane, was there to assist me, and I didn't stay out for long, but when I came to myself, I was unable to put any weight on my arms to push my body up or to pick up my briefcase. Marvin took my briefcase for me and helped me to my feet. We were heading to a hotel in Budapest to spend the night and would board a plane the next day for Albania.

Marvin and I had separate rooms at the hotel. He got me settled into my room and left. I was in much pain and had nearly no use of my hands, arms, etc. I did manage to call home and talk to Cherie about the situation. At that point, I did not know the extent of the injury to my arms, I just knew they were very painful and they were useless to me. I told her I felt that I should come back home and not go on to Albania because I had no idea if I would get worse or what to expect as far as getting any medical help in Albania.

Cherie did not give me the answer I was looking for, which was, "Just come on home, honey." Instead, she began to tell me that I needed to think that maybe Satan was doing all he could to keep me from going on to Albania and if I could manage to go at all, I should go. I listened to her and decided I would try to make it as planned, but I had a terrible night in the hotel. My arms hurt so badly I thought about getting into a tub of hot water and soaking them. I filled a deep, narrow European bathtub with hot water and got in, and it did feel good to put them in the water. However, when it was time to get out, I was totally helpless. I could not use my arms to pull myself up onto my knees or feet to get out of the tub. What a crazy mess I was in! The only thing I could do was use my toes to pull the plug out and let the tub drain completely dry, and then I was able to somehow get myself up and out. I had an impossible time brushing my teeth and shaving as well. Even turning on the faucet in the sink was a near impossibility. I had never been in such a helpless state. It was very painful to do anything at all with my arms. I must say, I was rethinking continuing on this journey.

I took plenty of ibuprofen and went to bed and slept. The next day, the only position that I could hold my arms that didn't give me great pain and throbbing was with my elbows bent and hands extended up, much like someone was holding a gun to my back. That is how I had to walk around and sit on the plane going to Albania. Thank God, it was only a two-hour flight.

When we arrived in Albania, some American missionaries met us and took me to the very best military hospital they had in the capital city of Tirana. This was when I got to know Hugh and Debbie Hoffman who were there working faithfully with Hope for the World. They were retired from our American military and were hard workers. Though the Albanian hospital was the best in the country, it was worse than anything you could imagine. It was very dirty with obsolete equipment. The doctors were smoking all over the hospital, and I saw blood on the bedding in some of the rooms where I looked. They had an antique World War II X ray machine in that hospital, and the doctor wanted to X ray my elbows. But the machine was locked up in a room, and they had to go out into the city to find the man at home who was the only one who had a key. They finally found him and got the room unlocked and took the X rays.

The film was on a tiny square that looked like an old 35 mm slide. I don't know how they could even see anything on it because it was so miniscule. They said it just looked like I had gotten contusions and had no breaks. They wrapped my arms and elbows and gave me some Tylenol and sent me on my way. By the way, when I got home and visited my doctor, I had cracked both elbows and was put into physical therapy for weeks.

To say that I had a difficult few days in Albania with my arms in this shape is a huge understatement, but I was so driven by what I was seeing. Somehow, I managed to go every day and view the work that was already being done and still needed to be done. The extreme poverty of this country and the lack of everything including vehicles, medical supplies, clothing, food, and drink made me totally forget about myself. Instead, I concentrated on how I might be used to bring help and hope to these suffering people in some way.

On the first day of my visit, I was taken to the school-age orphanage in Tirana where there were 170 children just barely existing in a four-story block building. It was cold weather, being in March, and yet they had no glass in the windows in most of the rooms, no heat in the building, and children were running everywhere in dirt and filth. The bathrooms were very unsanitary, with toilets that were simply square porcelain trough-like squares on the floor with a hole for the sewerage. There was a small dripping of water coming from a hose or pipe down the wall to help wash the waste down the hole. There was hardly any water pressure, so you can imagine the stench in these rooms. You talk about an experience using those things! Oh my goodness! This was the type of facilities that were present in most any public buildings and many homes at that time. Some were just cleaner than others, but that was the style. Turkish toilets, I believe, is what they were called. Definitely very difficult for people like me who had never used one. We jokingly dubbed them "squattie potties."

When I got to that orphanage and saw those kids and saw that they were living there with basically no decent food, heat, clothing, or beds to sleep on, my heart was broken! I could not believe what I was seeing. I just wanted to hurry through this mission trip and get back home and forget all of this and pray for them. That was what I thought I was going to take home with me from this trip—*a burden to pray.*

After spending several more days there and seeing more of the vast needs among not only the children at that particular orphanage but also visiting a baby orphanage where the babies were literally tied to their cribs, never being taken out and held, I was a mess emotionally. When I saw them rocking themselves back and forth in their rusty metal cribs, with not much of any milk in their bottles but a mixture of water and something else (cereal or vegetables), I was totally burdened and weeping and praying about what God would have me to do to help these poor little children.

I managed to live through that week and nearly forgot my own pain, although it was still there, and I knew my elbows and arms had swollen a lot. I could feel it. I am thankful that Marvin was traveling home with me too, so he could take care of my briefcase and help get my luggage through everywhere because I surely couldn't lift anything yet.

All the way home from Europe during the eighteen hours of travel, God kept speaking to my heart and telling me, "Roger, I need you to surrender to work as a missionary with Hope for the World and dedicate yourself to helping these orphans of Albania."

Well, I argued back and forth all of the way home about why I couldn't do it. I had no experience, I didn't know one thing about learning a foreign language, and I was too old to learn anyway. In fact, I was fifty-three years old and too old to start on such an adventure with my wife (who incidentally is three years older than I am). We were at an age in life where we should be looking toward a retirement of some type and trying to take it easy for the rest of our lives. After all, that's what most people do in their fifties and sixties in America.

I can tell you that by the time the plane landed in Atlanta, God had won all those arguments, and though I had no idea how it was going to work out, I had surrendered, locked, stocked, and barreled to take on this mission for Albanian orphans. Hope for the World had already been working there for nearly two years as an organization trying to repair the government orphanage building enough so they might begin to be able to heat it, etc. They were also helping with the provision of food for the children, warm blankets, etc. There was a man who was the director of the work in Albania, but he needed to resign and come back to the United States. It would then be my job to act in his place, stateside, collaborating between the American workers, the nationals, the orphan children, and the various government ministries, such as the Ministry of Labor and Ministry of Social Services. We wanted to provide the most effective assistance we could and at the same time bring a strong Christian testimony to this country and especially to these orphan children who had been raised in a Godless and atheistic society under the strong arm of communism all of their lives.

If I were to get involved in this ministry, I would have to coordinate work projects and find people to represent our interests in the orphan home, but mainly I would have to raise money here in America to send over there for food, clothing, and heat for these poor orphan children. I would also be in communication by email with the volunteers over there on a regular basis and try to develop a smooth-running machine. I guess my experience as a supervisor at the Milan Army Ammunition Plant years ago was coming into play once again. That was where I learned how to manage a group of people and get the best from them on their job. I'm thankful for that experience because I was truly overwhelmed by all that I saw and knew would have to be done in Albania and was definitely a rookie when it came to being a missionary.

When I got home and tried to tell Cherie all that had happened, I couldn't tell her without weeping, and she wept with me. That assured me that God had been preparing her heart as well. We agreed together with God that we would do all we could to make a difference in the lives of those suffering orphan children of Albania. We called Brother Jimmy Franks and told him we were *in* for the long haul, and we have been ever since. That was twenty-five years ago in March of 2019, and we are still busy and amazed at what God has been doing. We count it a real joy and privilege just to be a part of it all.

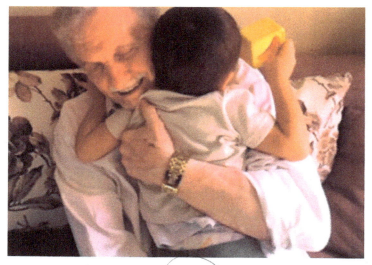

The orphan children were his calling…
They still have his heart after all these years.

Early Memories

By Perparim Demcellari

Perparim Demcellari is the in-country president of Hope for the World Albania. He is Albanian, and it has been our distinct joy and privilege to have this godly, wisdom-filled man on our staff since 1999. I had asked him to write some of his early memories concerning Hope for the World in Albania, and he was so gracious to do just that. I have taken just a little bit of editorial license in putting down his comments but have not tried to change the heart from which he has spoken. Here are words from Perparim:

I feel honored and at the same time obligated to somehow give my help and contribution to this book you are writing, Cherie. I began my service with Hope for the World in 1999, but my memories related to HFTW and especially to Brother Roger started in 1994.

In 1994, I was serving as an assistant pastor to missionary Pastor David Young, when we met with Brother Roger at the Young's apartment which was actually a part of the same building complex as the Tirana school-age orphanage at the time. I remember that Brother Roger had an accident coming to Albania and hurt his arms during his trip, and though he was in great pain, I could see his energies and his vitality as well as his deep burden for the country along with his great sense of humor. That day, I also found out that the reason for his trip to Albania was to determine the direction for HFTW in

Albania and what would be their role in the future and if they were going to have a permanent ministry in Albania or not.

On his second trip to Albania, I found out that Brother Roger had been made the director of HFTW for Albania. In a very funny way he said to me, "You wanted me to become the president of HFTW, and here I am, a director instead of president, so that's a done deal, but it's basically the same thing anyway!" And he laughed, and I did, too. Brother Roger took over the leadership in Albania for HFTW at that time. Once he took on this position, he brought new vision concerning all of the activities of HFTW in Albania, and he brought HFTW's reputation to high levels within the country.

My memories related to the Mullins family, and especially to Brother Roger, cannot be divided from the activity of HFTW in Albania. First, in sharing the gospel and winning souls and bringing them to God. Under HFTW's care and support, two churches were started in Albania, one in Tirana and one in Shkoder. Roger and Cherie would come to Albania and go to these specific churches. They would sing, play the piano, and share the message from the Bible. We were amazed and would listen to them very intently. They were so encouraging to these churches helping them spiritually as well as financially. They have also been a great encouragement and help to plant another church in the deepest village in north Albania, in Tropoje. I remember they also made trips to minister in other outlying mountain villages in Albania at various times.

The main focus of HFTW in Albania, however, was the orphans. Not just to help with humanitarian aid but to also provide spiritual food and Christian teaching for the orphan children. At each orphanage, HFTW started regularly scheduled Bible classes with the children every week. Because of this, hundreds of children have come to know Christ as their personal Savior.

Missionaries sent over through HFTW were the first to start sharing the gospel in the prisons as well. In order for that to happen, I had to get permission from the Albanian government. I personally had to intervene at the office of *General Directory for Prisons*. I also remember these missionaries sharing God's word with the Albanian dictator's widow. Yes, Enver Hoxha's wife, who was in prison at that time. I later was able to use this as a good argument for HFTW to not be limited only to prison ministry but to also share the gospel with the orphan children at the orphanages. It was at that time that they gave us a special room in each orphanage to carry out this activity, and that continues to this day.

Missionaries of HFTW were also the first ones who started sharing the gospel with the Gypsy community in Albania. They met with the leadership or the head of this community where they were selling used clothing. There is an outreach to the Gypsy people group in Albania today through HFTW staff members and other brothers and sisters in Christ who attend the churches mentioned earlier. Many in the Gypsy community have become Christians. There was also a time when HFTW-Romania brought a group of Gypsies from their country who had been saved. They came and stayed at our Tag Center and did an evangelistic outreach to the Roma (Gypsy) community near Tirana as they spoke the very same dialect. This was under the direction of HFTW missionary director to Romania, Tony Collicco. We were blessed to have them come to Albania.

Under Brother Roger's leadership, Hope for the World, Albania, which started first by helping the Zyber Hallulli Orphanage in Tirana, has now extended its outreach and commitment to three orphanages in Shkoder, one in Tirana, one in Korce, and one in Saranda, along with their aid to a special center for the handicapped in Shkoder and an elderly center in Saranda. In 2000, they began their first special center, *The Tag Center*, to help orphan children between the ages of fourteen to eighteen. I want to let you know why we named this facility The Tag Center. There is a very worthwhile story about this, and it deserves to be told. So I'll just take a little detour right here and allow Brother Fred Tag to tell the story of how this special place came to be."

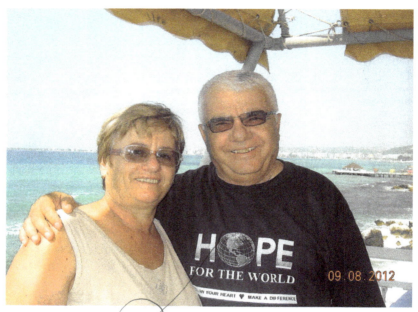

Perparim and Aferdlta Demcellari
Our In-Country President and his wife.

The Tag Center: Trek For Hope 2000

By Fred Tag

There's nothing more exciting in the life of a Christian than the time he accepts Christ and commits his life to serve him. I've heard this all my thirty-four plus years of serving our Lord, but I've recently concluded that that may not be a completely accurate statement. Accepting Jesus as Savior is exciting, but Jesus tells us that "I am come that they might have life, and that they might have it more abundantly" (John 10:10). There is much more to life than meets the eye, and the abundant life in Christ is not merely being well supplied in our physical needs. God intends to supply us with much, much more things that we have not even conceived of!

As I think back on my first experiences of serving God in Albania through Hope for the World, the joy that was experienced in and through that ministry parallels that of the salvation experience! I remember the calling to that ministry some twenty years ago like it was yesterday! I remember Bro. Roger Mullins giving a report to the church I was attending about a recent mission trip to Romania. At the end of that service, he shared the new ministry he had recently been called to, Hope for the World, a ministry to orphans in the country of Albania. Well there is always the likelihood that by lunchtime the following day, little that the missionary said the previous day would be resting on my mind. However, on this occasion, I could not get my mind off those children on the other side of the world! In fact, the emotional weight that I experienced only got heavier with each following day. After three weeks of debating with God as to what to do with this weight, I finally went to my pastor and sought counsel as to how to handle my feelings. Long story short, after a short time of conversation with Bro. Roger, I found myself planning my first mission trip to the country of Albania.

As an airline employee by profession, I was very comfortable with domestic travel, but when the reality hit that I was traveling halfway across the world to a third-world country, the butterflies started working overtime! When the day finally came to board the airplane, I truly wondered what in the world I had gotten myself into. Back in those days, an airline employee had to travel as if he were attending Sunday morning services, a suit and tie was a must. I remember Bro. Roger commenting that the Albanians would assume that I was some sort of important millionaire by virtue of my formal dress. I laughed at the goofy comment, but little did I know that after five minutes of exiting the airplane at the Tirana airport, I felt like a billionaire in comparison to those around me. It was not a good feeling! For the first time in my life, any resemblance of a need in my life was completely blown away by those living in true poverty and truly in need!

The purpose of this mission trip was simply to observe and experience the ministry of Hope for the World in Albania and to follow God to whatever he might have me do to help the ministry and these orphan children. As an amateur photographer, one small contribution I could make on this trip was to take pictures of the orphans in order to make sponsorship packets for distribution back in the United States with the intent to gain supporters or sponsors. I remember walking into that orphan home on the first day in Albania, trying to take pictures of children while tears streamed down my face! The conditions that I found these innocent children living in completely took me off guard! There was no doubt; I had to do whatever I could to help these little ones! I told people I had 302 kids—two here in the United States that live in my home and three hundred in Albania!

Over the next few years, I spent time doing whatever Bro. Roger and the Holy Spirit deemed necessary in an effort to further the ministry in Albania. From gathering toothbrushes for these children to presenting the ministry to churches, I was open to whatever the Lord had in mind.

At the same time, I was closing in on middle age. With all the business of life, I felt I had to do something to keep physically active. Running was difficult due to knee issues, so I decided to take up cycling as it was actually beneficial for my knees! As with most everything I seem to get involved with, I tend to push things to the extreme. As time progressed, short bicycle rides evolved into longer rides, with the occasional one hundred-mile "century" organized ride. I even heard of crazy people riding their bicycles across America, from coast to coast! While on these long bicycle rides, one has plenty of time to think and pray! While riding and thinking, once again, the Holy Spirit began to plant seeds that seemed to sprout no matter how hard I tried to ignore them. Could I actually ride my bicycle across the United States to help orphan children in Albania?

As I began to piece the logistics of a coast-to-coast bicycle ride together in my mind, the more I realized the impossibility of such a venture! From taking five weeks away from my job to raising the funds to make it all worthwhile, it just didn't seem likely! On top of all that, the looks I got from people (notably my dear wife, Debbie, and Roger and Cherie, to mention a few) when I mentioned the plan that was churning in the back of my mind were priceless. I'm convinced they thought I had totally lost my mind! It really didn't make a lot of sense to me either! But, once again, God would not let my mind rest. In an effort to finally put this ridiculous idea to rest, I decided to attempt the first and largest obstacle, getting five straight weeks off from my job as a supervisor at a major airline! The thought of my boss finding a way to let me go for that long was just not going to happen! But then it dawned on me, my boss was an avid cyclist too! When I explained that I wanted to raise money for poor little orphan kids, and do it on a bicycle, his response was, "Sounds great, we'll somehow just make it happen!" I was shocked!

Getting enough time away from my job was one thing, but raising the funds to make it all worthwhile was another! I figured that if I could raise $10,000 above the cost to support the trip, then it would be a worthwhile project to pursue. Such a fund-raising venture would require some out-of-the box thinking. It would require involvement of more people than I or my church could gather together! I decided to call on a new friend of mine, Rick Davison, station manager at J93.3 Christian radio, to see if he could help with a listener-supported fund-raiser. I remember that day like it was yesterday! Roger and I pitched the idea of a three thousand-mile coast-to-coast bicycle trip to raise money for Hope for the World orphans. My basic plan was to ask individuals to support me with a penny for every mile I rode, times three thousand miles, or simply thirty dollars for the entire trip. Rick's reply was, "If I could get one thousand listeners to support you a penny per mile, that would be about thirty thousand dollars, how would that be?" After literally breaking down in tears, I gathered myself together and acknowledged that this was truly an answer to prayer! At that moment, I realized that "Trek for Hope 2000" would become a reality! I was quickly learning that when God is in it, he will make a way!

For the next year and nine months, I spent most of my spare time planning and fund-raising! The more I thought about all that would be required to pull off a coast-to-coast bicycle trip, the more I realized that I had my hands full! From acquiring spare bicycle parts to writing letters, scheduling and attending fund-raising events, not to mention hours of physical training, there was a lot to be done! I presented the event to many churches, businesses, friends, and family. The details seemed endless, but God continued to open doors that I couldn't have opened myself! There was no turning back!

When I mentioned the whole idea to my pastor, Chuck Holt, of Fairview Baptist Church, I was surprised to learn that not only did he think it was a great idea, but he wondered if I would like to have a riding partner. Certainly, the three thousand-mile journey would be much more enjoyable with some company, so I openly welcomed the idea! Another unlikely addition to the crew was my uncle, Charles Mowry. Uncle Charlie signed on as commander in chief of the support crew, but at age seventy-two, he decided to ride some of the way also!

After much planning, training, and praying, the last few days prior to the beginning of Trek for Hope 2000 came quickly! A very promising J93.3 radio telethon yielded almost $33,000 in pledges, not to mention another $20 plus thousand generated through local churches and personal contacts! All we had to do now was to ride our bicycles a mere three thousand miles! The trip would begin in Monterey, California, and end at Tybee Island in Savannah, Georgia. Since Monterey was my brother's hometown, I was thankful that Paul and his wife, Becky, had coordinated the commencement of the trip on the west coast! With Uncle Charles and the support vehicle in place in Monterey, my pastor, myself, and my family boarded a plane for Monterey.

Finally, the day had come! On May 13, a crowd had gathered at the seashore where we would ceremonially dunk our rear tires in the Pacific Ocean, signifying the beginning of this very long journey! The first day of our trip proved to be our longest, from Monterey to Pasa Robles! For a good portion of that first leg, I was blessed to have my brother, Paul, and his wife, Becky; my wife, Debbie; and our children, Heather and Aaron. We were also very blessed to have Robin Brody, Paul's friend and avid cyclist, with us for the entire first day! Robin rode with us and took on the burden of navigating that first day! After about fifty miles of riding, the entire crew shared a picnic lunch together. It was a classy spread put together by Paul and Becky, followed by what I had been dreading, a hug and kiss from my family whom I would not see again for another four weeks! We arrived in Pasa Robles that evening with just a few minutes of daylight to spare. After peddling 120 miles, we were safe, tired, and glad the first day was behind us!

As the sun rose the next morning, we grabbed a quick breakfast and prepared to do it all over again! This day, however, it would be just Chuck and me, along with Uncle Charles and our support vehicle driver for the first week. As we said goodbye to Robin, who was peddling back to Monterey, we continued our trek eastward with the Atlantic Ocean as our final destination!

I'll spare you the amazing details of the seemingly endless hours of peddling a bicycle through the California desert! The route I had planned would basically follow Interstate 40 which takes the southern route across the country. What got old really fast was the fact that the first five days and five hundred miles would be spent in the very large state of California. The excitement of peddling for days through the windy, sandy, and near one hundred-degree desert temperatures is simply more than I care to convey! I'm not sure if "brownout" is a valid term, but it seems to be the only way to describe the day we rode through a desert sandstorm, with visibility at one hundred feet or less! After five days and five hundred plus miles, the "Welcome to Arizona" sign was a sight for sore eyes!

With California in our rearview mirror, a renewed hope that progress was being made energized us! Unfortunately, that energy would be spent peddling up a very large hill, climbing almost seven thousand feet from Needles, California, to the Continental Divide in a span of four days. Up until now, our average speed was somewhere between sixteen to eighteen mph on flat terrain. As we began to climb, our speed dipped down to ten to twelve mph range, with the steepest portions dropping to the seven to eight mph range. If you do the math, this four hundred-mile stretch turned out to be the longest and toughest portion of our journey!

With every ounce of heart, mind, and soul committed to peddling uphill for four straight days, the giant sign on I-40 that read "Continental Divide" brought the realization that the uphill battle was over, at least for now! As we started to descend from that point, what a welcome change! Instead of an average speed of nine mph, we were now experiencing speeds of twenty-five to thirty mph. Not only that, we were working half as hard to accomplish those speeds. Our legs were in desperate need for a semi-relaxed pace for the next few days!

Speaking of body parts, by now after nine to ten days of riding, there were certain parts of my body that were beginning to talk to me! My legs were hanging in there, and basically the rest of my body was getting used to eight to ten hours a day on a bicycle. There was one part, however, that began to give me great concern! It was the main contact point between the bicycle and the body, the seat! Now, in an effort to keep things polite, let's just say that things were beginning to wear on me! If you watched professional cyclists on TV, or even on the local streets, you'll notice the tight-fitting aerodynamic shorts they are wearing. The main function of these shorts is to provide padding in critical areas to cushion the ride. I was at the point that extra cushion became a dire necessity! Extra cushion meant wearing an extra pair of cycling shorts. After this minor adjustment, let's just say that things began to smooth out!

As we pressed forward on our five-week journey, every day was an adventure! From sandstorms to rainstorms, there were days that it became more than just a little uncomfortable to be riding long distance on a bicycle! But those days were peppered with blessings. With media attention via K-Love Radio and limited TV coverage, there were the occasional individuals that somehow heard of our venture and recognized us at a rest stop or at our final destination for the day! The donations and words of encouragement reenergized us, and being reminded of the cause went far in easing the pain of those long days in the saddle!

As we pressed eastward, our downhill stretch from the Continental Divide eventually leveled out. Long flat stretches of road were replaced with rolling hills as we peddled through Texas, Oklahoma, and Arkansas! When possible, we enjoyed traveling back in time as we traveled through many old abandoned towns via Route 66. I could vividly see in my mind a young couple enjoying a root beer float as they cruised the streets of their tiny town. My imagination was short-lived as a pattern of peddling up and down the hills brought me back to reality! We would peddle to the top of one hill and down the other side, only to find another hill was waiting. Hill after hill, they seemed to never end! It was like winning a battle only to find that there was yet another waiting in the wings! The scenery also began to change as we transitioned from the dry desert to a milder greener climate. Everything seemed to be in slow motion! At the end of each day, our impression of each town where we stayed for the night largely depended on the quality of the showerhead and the comfort of the bed for the night!

There were other distractions that would keep us entertained as the miles passed by. Mooing to the grazing cows as we peddled by their pasture and trying to hold our breath as long as possible when we peddled by the poor armadillo roadkill were just a few. Then there was that one exciting Sunday afternoon as we rolled through a quiet little town. As we approached the outskirts, we could see the excitement that was evident by virtue of the flashing blue lights of law enforcement! The police cars were slowly approaching with some sort of commotion between us and the blue lights. As we approached, it all came into focus. A small herd of goats were being herded by the city's finest! As we slowly peddled by, to our amazement and apparently attracted to our colorful apparel, the goats began to chase us! Boy, can those little guys run! As we were clearly bringing chaos to this quiet afternoon, law enforcement ordered us to stop! Apparently, a search was being conducted as to where these rogue vigilantes belonged. Finally, things had calmed down to the point that the police released us for good behavior!

The journey was filled with ups and downs, but none was more memorable than the day of June 4. It was midday, and we had just crossed over the Mississippi River. What an amazing sight as we peddled across the Helena Bridge from Arkansas to Mississippi! Once across the river, we noticed that the paved shoulder that we enjoyed riding on most of our trip had disappeared. Over the last three weeks, there were few times that we felt really uncomfortable having to share the road with motor vehicles. This particular stretch of road had us on edge. We had nowhere to ride but to the left of the white line on the edge of the narrow two-lane highway! We peddled a very uncomfortable six miles before turning south on Route 61, a four-lane highway still with no shoulder to ride on. The good news was that there was little to no traffic, with lots of room for motor vehicles to pass in the left lane. But then came that Red S-10 pickup! I was leading at this particular moment as my pastor and I would take turns playing follow the leader! As Chuck noticed the approaching vehicle, he also noticed that it appeared to be heading right for us! At the last second, to avoid being hit, Chuck left the roadway and crashed his bicycle into brush on the side of the highway. Unfortunately for me, I had no time to react. The S-10 struck my bicycle, slamming me into the sharp gravel on the shoulder of the highway! The truck that hit me never even stopped! After the police report was completed, a trip to the Northwest Mississippi Regional Medical Center was in order! Thankfully, there were no broken bones! A healthy case of road rash covered the left side of my body, and a prescription for Darvocet would help mask the pain over the next few days. My very expensive bicycle was destroyed, but fortunately, I had brought a spare that was neatly tucked away in the cargo compartment of the support vehicle! My spare Cannondale bicycle would have to take me the rest of the way, if I was able! Fortunately, June 5 was a scheduled rest day! It was a day that both Chuck and I needed to collect our thoughts and evaluate our situation! With only eight more days of riding to complete the journey, the thought of throwing in the towel was one option to seriously consider!

In spite of our miserable physical condition, and a renewed appreciation of life itself, we decided to press on! My pastor was nursing an injured shoulder, and I was trying to not take any pain meds with the idea that drugs and cycling probably don't mix very well!

At this point, you might be thinking this had to be the hardest part of the trip! Quite honestly, I have to admit, it was very difficult for me to get back on the bicycle for fear of what was approaching from behind! However, there was something that I had been dealing with for the last three weeks that I had not expected. The absolute hardest part of this venture was missing my wife and children. I remember times when even though I was exhausted from the daily one hundred-mile ride, I couldn't rest or sleep due to longing to see my family! Missing my family hurt in a way that I had never experienced!

Most of the miles were behind us now, and finally the day had come that we would ride into our hometown on the south side of Atlanta. There was a big welcome party planned at our home church, Fairview Baptist of Jonesboro, Georgia. Even though our journey wasn't complete, it was the light at the end of the tunnel. Seeing my family and spending a short weekend with them were the medicine I needed to cure my homesickness! We were on the home stretch!

On Monday, June 12, we departed from Jonesboro for the remaining 281 miles that would take us to Tybee Island beach in Savannah. It was one of the hottest legs of the trip, with temperatures well over one hundred degrees. Ironically, it happened to also be one of the coldest, when a windy rainstorm had us soaked, shivering, and taking cover at an abandoned gas station. On June 14, we rolled into Savannah where another church welcomed us with a night of celebration and TV news coverage! The following morning, we rode a short eighteen miles to complete our journey as we dunked our front tires in the Atlantic Ocean! What an amazing experience, God had seen us through!

God had accomplished something through the lives of Fred Tag and Chuck Holt, something that I never thought possible. God had provided strength, courage, and finances for orphan children that would change their lives, and ours, forever. J93.3 radio had collected an unprecedented near 100 percent of the money that was pledged during the Trek for Hope Radiothon, and the entire project yielded over $58,000!

For me, the impact on children halfway around the world would not totally be realized until some five years later. Due to circumstances beyond my control, I was unable to make the trip to Albania to see the fruits of all those peddled miles until 2005. The money generated from Trek for Hope 2000 was well spent on renovating a building that would provide shelter to older orphan kids beyond the government-provided orphan homes. Hope for the World named it The Tag Center for Teens. What an honor! Words can't describe how I felt when I saw the sign hanging over the door of that building! I was even further touched by the welcome party and the testimonies of the orphans themselves of how God had changed their lives through Hope for the World and The Tag Center.

I would like to conclude with just a few thoughts. First, I must make one thing clear! Fred Tag had accomplished little, but God had accomplished everything! I had learned several valuable lessons!

1. I experienced firsthand Matthew 19:26 that says: "But, Jesus beheld them, and said unto them, 'With men this is impossible; but with God all things are possible'."

2. I learned that when God leads us into action, he can accomplish great things through a willing heart.
3. I realized that God not only used two middle-aged guys riding bicycles but hundreds of willing souls that believed, gave, and followed a vision!

It would be impossible for me to mention all those who had a part in Trek for Hope 2000. But I would like to say a special thanks to the following people who went above and beyond to make it all possible:

Roger and Cherie Mullins, for their faith and support.

My family, Debbie, Heather, and Aaron Tag, for their loving support and doing without Dad.

Pastor Chuck Holt, for being my riding buddy.

My uncle, Charles Mowry, our support vehicle commander who, at age seventy-two, rode his bicycle over six hundred miles.

Rick Davison and crew, for the J93.3 Radiothon.

Paul and Becky Tag, for organization on the west coast.

Tom Grimes, Fred Upchurch, Jimmy Fischer, George Blake, and Paul Tag, for driving the support vehicle.

And the three hundred plus orphans in Albania whose need taught me many things and brought me closer to God through his amazing love and grace!

Perparim Continues

Because the Tag Center was government-owned, it became apparent that HFTW needed to have their own property in order to carry out their work effectively. In 2010, that became a reality with our "Hope Center" located in Marikaj. We are happy to say that out of the teens who have come through the Tag Center and Hope Center, 40 percent of them have gone on to the university. After leaving our centers, they are assisted to become well integrated into life. The contribution of HFTW to the orphan children in Albania has been extraordinary in providing food, clothing, and other important needs for their education and living conditions.

Through the years, HFTW has also been of great assistance to the orphanages and their facilities by providing reconstruction, repairs, maintenance, building playgrounds, and sports fields for the children. I remember at times in the earlier years when military planes from Dobbins AFB in Atlanta, Georgia, were provided to HFTW through the Denton Amendment on a number of occasions. They were loaded with food, appliances, supplies, clothing, and all kinds of materials and needs for the children as well as the churches and missionaries within the country. (Editor's note: Hope for the World was asked one time to bring a complete set of the "GA Code Annotated," and a judge from Atlanta was kind enough to donate this to Albania to assist them in setting up the laws to govern their people.)

Through HFTW, the conditions of the orphanages changed radically from horrible to good. It has been HFTW's loving care that has brought so much happiness to the children as well as the workers in the orphanages through the celebration of birthdays, Christmas, Easter, Orphans Day, Children's Day, and Independence Day. On these special days, HFTW provides the financial support to take the children on excursions to different cities of Albania or just a short field trip of some type within their own city. It is through HFTW that the lives of these poor orphan children have been changed and been made more colorful, much happier, and generally more enriched. HFTW has truly been making a difference in their lives.

There are many other humanitarian projects that have been conducted in Albania by HFTW. During the Kosovo crisis in 1999, HFTW was there to help in many ways with food, transportation, and care. The orphans were baking hundreds of loaves of bread each day at the orphanage and carrying them to the refugee camps in the Tirana area.

HFTW also plays a strong role in the lives of orphan teens who have had to leave the orphanages and move to the government tech dorms or onto the streets. We have helped these young people with many personal needs and supplies. Aid has also been provided for orphaned children within other villages surrounding Tirana. During a flood in Shkoder, HFTW was there to help families in the area through distributing food, clothes, etc.

In regard to our reputation within the country of Albania, in 1996, per instructions from Brother Roger, together with the help of Pastor David Young, we worked over the legislation concerning the court decision for the activity of HFTW in Albania. We are highly respected by the Albanian government, and we are careful to honor all of our relationships with the various ministries with which we work and with the orphanages by executing contracts concerning each facility with which we are involved in the country. Because we abide by their laws, and due to the positive experience and contribution of HFTW through the years, we have been granted two licenses. We are licensed to do our activities in helping the community and to operate the orphanages. Then, more recently, we have been granted the license for the right of HFTW to own and operate its own center, the Hope Center in Marikaj, Albania.

I really appreciate the ministry of HFTW and especially the hard work of Roger and Cherie Mullins who have been directors in Albania since 1994. They have been solely responsible for raising the money to care for Albanian orphans and the elderly. I know how hard they have to work to raise these funds, but I also know what a wonderful group of Christian people in America have been there sponsoring children for years and years and giving over and above their own tithes with special offerings to God through this organization. I cannot praise God enough for all that has been accomplished with this huge group of believers who have wanted to make an impact on the future of Albania through the orphan children.

When we first began with this work in 1994, banks did not exist in many towns in Albania. I had to carry cash to our directors in Shkoder and Saranda. These locations are hours away from Tirana and our home office. Now things have improved in our country, and we can wire from bank to bank. The wonderful thing is that 100 percent of all money given for the orphan children goes totally to the orphan children and not to the administration of these orphanages. It is our staff that does every bit of the shopping for the needs of the orphan children.

Through the years, I have seen so many wonderful mission teams sent over here through HFTW. These groups would come from churches in America and would be such a blessing and help with different projects at the orphanages in Tirana, Shkoder, Saranda, Vlore, and Korce. Other special missionaries have also started a life here in Albania and live here with us. They are giving amazing help and training to the Albanian staff and bringing about a different mentality. At the Hope Center, we have an American missionary lady, Pam Arney, from Georgia. She has been in Albania now for a number of years. She is a great help in our work at the Hope Center and with the teens and our staff.

I am happy to express gratitude to HFTW in Albania on behalf of the orphan children, directors of the orphanages, staff of HFTW, government officials, and other leaders of our country. "Certificates of Appreciation" and many "Thank You" plaques have been presented to Brother Roger and HFTW through the years from various groups. One very special moment was when the City Fathers honored him in Shkoder as a "Citizen of Honor."

I was truly blessed to be able to contribute this portion to your book, Cherie. Thank you so much for inviting me to have a part. I wish you every success.

God bless you,

Perparim Demcellari, Albanian President
Hope for the World, Albania

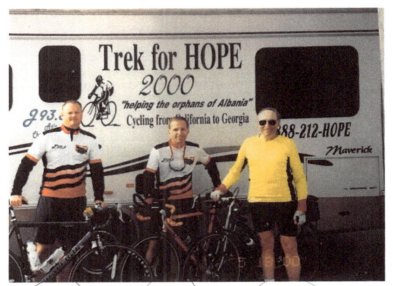

Fred Tag (center) Chuck Holt (left), Uncle Charlie (right)

Those Howard Boys

In March of 1994, when we began our work with the Albanian orphans, our grandsons, Brady and Austin Howard, born to our daughter, Cindy, and her husband, Andy Howard, were very much a part of our everyday lives in Henry County, Georgia. At that time, Brady (B) was five years old, and Austin (A) was one year old. Those were the nicknames Poppy (Roger) gave them, just simply A and B. We had so much fun with those two little guys! We were really thankful they were in our world because when our son, Buddy, and his wife, Kerri, moved off to Nashville, it left a great big empty spot, since we had never been separated from Buddy before. But I kid you not, it was absolutely no problem *at all* for Brady and Austin to crawl into that empty spot and fill it full to the brim with so many wonderful things.

Brady at that time was already beginning kindergarten at Fairview Elementary School, and we found ourselves on the front row cheering him on in any and all programs in which he was involved at the school. It was always fun as we were jammed in among all of the other grandparents, with our cameras, both video and regular, to get the first glimpse of him coming in, taking his place on stage to sing, or play his part in the Thanksgiving play or whatever other production he was in. I can remember how his father Andy would get up and stand against the wall with the video camera so that no one else would get in front of him in order to capture the very best coverage of the events. Oh, how well Brady would perform and play his starring roles! Well, at least to us he was always the star. Grandparents'

Day was always great at their schools. Sitting down for lunch with Brady and all his little rowdy friends was a real experience!

Brady was a lot of fun and a hard worker at a young age. His daddy made sure of that. In fact, back when he was just learning to walk, when they were building a house for his Paw Paw and Granny Howard, I can still see little Brady following Andy around with his tool belt dragging around his little waist, finding the nails his dad just pounded and giving them some extra taps with his trusty little rubber hammer. He reminded me of a Christian song I've heard before entitled, "Daddy, I Wanna Be Just Like You."

Another family video we have recently uncovered showed Andy having little Brady (all of about two years old) dragging his own car seat through the house on Sunday morning, getting ready to go to church. Andy started the work ethic in his boys at a very early age! Sometimes, we grandparents thought it was a bit much, but I can see today where it has truly paid off. Neither one of the Howard boys is afraid of hard work and is usually among the first to volunteer. Even if they didn't volunteer when they were young, their daddy made sure they were there on every work day at the church and part of many other jobs that required a lot of time and energy. We cannot claim one iota of credit for teaching them in this area, but we sure are glad that God gave us Andy as a son-in-law and as their dad.

Brady didn't play T-Ball as a little fellow; I don't really recall the reason. Maybe Andy just wasn't into T-Ball much at that time and didn't see a need for him to be an assistant coach. But Brady did start playing in the Henry County Youth Recreational Baseball League when he was about seven or eight years old. You can be sure that as soon as he was suited up and on the team, all four of us grandparents were there to see every game we could! Bob and "Sweet Pea" Howard have been our lifelong friends, even before Cindy and Andy began to date. It's so much fun sharing "in-law" responsibilities with them! We grandparents tried to make it to every game we could, and we did get to most of them! I can assure you, Brady always had a great cheering section whenever he took the bat in his hand. This was especially fun for us as it was a "first" in our lives. I can vividly remember holding umbrellas over our heads or running for cover at rainy-day games.

No matter what, we were always there along with Bob and Sweet Pea or, as the boys called us, Poppy and Grammy and Paw Paw and Granny.

Watching sports activities was a new experience for Roger and me. You see, with our lifestyle through the years of evangelism, neither Buddy nor Cindy was able to participate in any sports programs like this, so we were actually feeling like some of the parents were with a first child on a team. Andy was nearly always a part of the coaching staff for any of the teams on which the boys played, and Cindy was a wonderful supporter, playing her role well in all of the "booster clubs" and in whatever ways it is that moms help with these teams. She spent many hours at the concession stand and, in later years, prepared chili or other crock pot meals for football teams. I can remember that sometimes she'd volunteer to head it up, which meant getting some of the other mothers to participate and volunteer for various fund-raisers and functions supporting the team. I always wondered how she did all of that and held down a full-time job and sang in the choir at Glen Haven Baptist Church, but she somehow managed. Even the other day, I found myself scratching my head and wondering how in the world she managed to be involved in so many things.

About the time Brady was on his first baseball team in the "Rec League," Austin was getting signed up for T-Ball. Now, this was something very entertaining to watch! These little guys were not much more than about five years old and had coaches working with them weekly, trying to teach them the very beginnings of baseball. I couldn't believe that they actually went to practice for this because when I went to a game, it looked to me like none of them had ever played before!

I can remember watching Austin play outfield on the team and instead of having his glove on his hand ready to catch a ball if it should come his way, he had his glove on his head and was going around in circles. And quite often, he'd have to look for his mommy to take him to potty! Oh what fun and how cute he was as a little slugger in his red and white uniform. Austin felt just as big as, if not bigger than, his brother Brady.

Paw Paw (Brother Bob) Howard, the boys' paternal grandfather, had bought a small wagon for Brady when he was just a little guy, and he had a special license plate made for the wagon that said "Bro. Brady." Bob always called him Brother Brady from his earliest days. Do you think he may have the gift of prophecy? It certainly is pretty amazing that Brady is now in full-time ministry and on our church staff and a true "Brother" Brady or "Pastor" Brady." Interesting, huh? On the other hand, one of the earliest photos of Austin was made of him posing with a *Wall Street Journal* opened in his hands, and he seems to be heading for the business world today. At the time I am writing this segment, Austin has graduated from college and is employed by J. R. Bowman Construction Company as a supervisor on some pretty impressive municipal buildings in a neighboring town right now. I also happen to know that on this coming Friday night, he will be proposing to a beautiful young lady named Suzanne Hembree who just happens to be the sister of Savannah Hembree who is married to Brady. So we are going to have the brothers married to sisters and sharing the same in-laws.

In Brady's early years, one of our gifts to him would quite often be a guitar. He has had everything from the tiniest "toy" guitars that you just push buttons and play to all the appropriate sizes as he grew. We even tried to introduce toy pianos and keyboards to him, but I think his dad frowned on that quite a bit, thinking we might make a "sissy-boy" piano player out of him. It looked to us like sports was going to win out over music with Brady for a long time, but there came a day when he actually wanted a "good" guitar. and his parents made sure he got one for Christmas one year. From that day on, we've watched him make his own choices in that area. We have seen that guitars and music have played a great role in Brady's life as he intertwines his music with his ministry on a regular basis. He put together a great group of young men as a praise band called "Finally Breathing" at our church. They are a real blessing to the youth in our area and in other churches. They are great additions to the summer camps, and we all enjoy them in our services at Glen Haven quite often.

I remember when Austin was just a little tyke, we wondered if he was ever going to talk. It seemed like he never spoke a word, and Brady never quit talking! In fact, we all felt that Austin just let Brady be his spokesperson, and guess what, Brady enjoyed it because that kid never met a stranger and talked to everyone, young and old alike. When Austin did begin to speak, he had a little slush in his speech which required some speech therapy, but it was soon remedied, and you'd never know it now.

Austin was always the quiet one in the family, but then there were certain things about him that made me wonder about what went on in that little head of his because they say that "still waters run deep." I'm thinking of so many times when he would be at my house, and when it came time for him to have a drink of something, he always wanted to use my little crystal stemware glasses that I used for fruit juice. He'd want something like grape juice in it, and he'd act like he was "drinking" wine like he'd seen on TV commercials or on the movie screen. I would think, *Oh, me, I hope this little guy isn't making a role model out of the drinking crowd*, and I'd pray extra hard for Austin. Ha ha.

Even though he started out being a very quiet child, when he did begin to talk, he sort of caught up, and I can remember going to his kindergarten room at school and seeing where he had to be reprimanded a few times for talking *too much* to all his little neighbors in the classroom. He was overly friendly to his friends, I guess. And with both of his grandfathers being preachers, what could we expect? In fact, one great thing I recall about Austin as a little guy, as he grew up in elementary and middle school at Eagles Landing Christian Academy, was that he liked to have Bible study groups with his friends. And he would quite often preach the sermon. He would collect ideas, thoughts, sermons, and even visual aids from his preacher grandfathers.

I'll never forget the night Poppy introduced him to his own sermon on "The Tater Family." When I told him we actually had a family that we had made out of Mr. Potato Heads and that each one was dressed to go with their name, and that they had their own traveling case and we still had it in our outbuilding, why you'd have thought we'd offered him a million dollars! He was so excited and wanted to meet the Tater Family. And though we hadn't had them out in years since we'd come off the road of evangelism, they were still safe and sound and in pretty good shape actually. That night, Austin met Daddy Dick Tater, Momma Agi-Tater, Brother Spec-Tater, Sister Common-Tater, Aunt Imi Tater, Uncle Ro Tater, and Cousin Hesi Tater. You can sort of figure out the sermon based on their names. Austin was one excited boy when he went out the door that night carrying their wooden motel box where they had been stored for so many years. These are some of the things we would do to entertain our grandchildren when they came to visit at our home.

Of course, things were not "super spiritual" around our house all the time. I will never forget, for instance, how many times I came into the living room and saw Poppy, Brady, and Austin pitching their dirty socks up at the ceiling fan to see how far each one would fling! I'd wonder if they'd ever find them again or if it would be Grammy to search them out and get them into the next load of laundry.

Now, you didn't think there was ever a chance that Austin and Brady wouldn't be talkers and entertainers, did you? They have entertained the whole family for years with their stories of everyday life as we gather around the table on special occasions. The Howard family has some deep-rooted family traditions, and Austin is the one who wants to make sure we keep all of them and invent more as we go through life. He is a real family traditionalist, which is very endearing.

I have kept an essay Austin wrote while in middle school. We were so proud of him not just for writing this good essay but because he wrote from his heart. I hope you'll enjoy. You can tell he is a deep thinker.

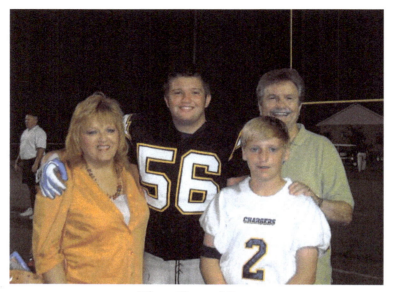

Those Howard Boys
Brady with his brother Austin and
Grammy and Poppy after one of ELCA's games.

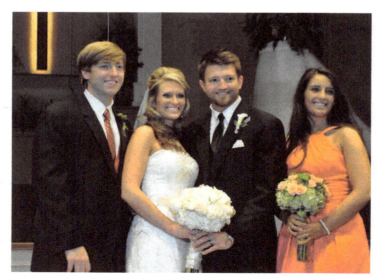

Those Howard Boys
Brady and Savannah's Wedding Day in 2013. Five years later, his brother Austin (left) is Marrying her sister Suzanne (right}.

This I Believe

By Austin Howard

This I believe, in a traditional society rather than the contemporary one in which we live in today. A society in which a kid can walk to school or to a friend's house, or even to the movies, and the parents have the peace of mind in knowing that their child will be safe. I believe in a society where the average Joe that walks the streets has his pants at his waist and his hat in the correct position. I believe in a father's hard work ethic in which he is able to be the breadwinner for the home and not have to depend upon the mother's income to help put food on the table. I also believe that a kid should be taught how to do work outside the house and manual labor which prepares him for life, where he will have to work his butt off to survive and succeed, rather than a child who is given everything and sits at home on the weekend inside playing video games, only hurting himself in the long term. I believe that a child's home should be his/her stronghold in which they can go to their parents about anything and not have the pressure of keeping hidden secrets which their friends know but their parents don't. I believe in music that doesn't have to say a cuss word every other word to be fun and enjoyable. I believe that if a male/female can wear slacks or a skirt to school, a funeral, a wedding, or even a party, then he/she should have the desire to want to look their best when they step into the Lord's house. I believe in the desire and passion of a Christian mother and father to press their children to become closer to the Lord, not letting them sleep in on Sundays or miss church for sports activities (I myself played travel baseball growing up and was not allowed to play on Sundays; at the time I hated it, but looking back upon it, I'm glad to call my parents godly Christians who always wanted and continue to want the best for my Christian walk). I believe in a church that doesn't have to conform to the world's appearance, and I believe that as Christians, we are called to be different and told by God that we will have to face trials and tribulations, but through Christ's strength, we can overcome them and grow closer to him each day. I believe in hymnals, for they are the true lyrical masterpieces made by warriors of the faith to bring honor and glory to our father, not like today's singers in which they imitate secular groups just so they can go "platinum" and make earthly wealth. I believe in a traditional American society; I also believe that I was born in the wrong era. I wish and dream every day that I was born in my parent's era or even my grandparent's in which I could attain all these desires. But I also believe that God has a plan for me and my life, and I believe that I was born in this generation for a purpose, and that purpose was to keep the traditional morals and values of the past strong throughout the generations to come. This is what I believe, that a traditional society is a lost treasure, only to be rediscovered through the lives of others like myself.

—Austin

Brady had quite a gift for literature and composition. Even as a young boy, in grammar school, he had an extremely active imagination and quite a vocabulary. Often, I would get to see some of his writings. Realizing that Brady was eight years old when he wrote this one, I think you'll get a kick out of it. I asked Brady if he minded if I included it in my book. He graciously approved. Thank you, Brady.

THE MAKING OF A WONDERFUL LIFE

> Brady (10) 2-3-98
>
> If I had a 100 Dollar Bill. I would go and get a limazeen, I'd fly to hollywood get into show biss. Then by a man chen, Have lunch with Bill Clinton, Buy a nitendo 64, Get a swimming pool, buy a big base ball feild, and buy a basket ball court, I'd then go back to hollywood start on my next movie "Young James Bond 007 Cats Are Very Jentle". Then I'd go and have a cup of tea with Mrs. Clinton. But even though I might have ran out of my first hundred dollar bill from the movies I'd have tons of them. Then go to dirt bike practice with the best dirt biker in the nation. Then practice football with The Bronko's. I'd finally at the end of the day get in my hot tub. I would go to Howard Indestries the next morning come home practice my movie have a tallar make me my clothes so the next morning I'll have some clothes to wear to work. That's what I'd Do.
> THE END

Brady's $100 Essay

I had a nice collection of nutcrackers that I would set out every Christmas. From the time Austin was a little fella, he was very interested in this collection. He couldn't wait to see where I was going to line them up each year. As he got big enough, he would help me unpack them, and if any of them needed some super glue anywhere, he would help put them in good shape. He has always had a mind to work and been a great helper. He was good at stringing lights all over my music room for Christmas, too. All kids love Christmas, but Austin really "got into" preparing for it. He still does that at the Howard Farm for that matter, where they have acres to decorate, not just a room or two.

Poppy loved to play "Paper, Scissors, Rocks" with both of the boys over and over again to pass the time with them! They loved that game, too. Of course, Roger has always been one to dress up in crazy outfits from time to time and entertain with his singing program on special occasions. Austin was always the one who wanted to dress up like him. They smiled with their "Bubba Teeth" and donned their funny hats and entertained all of the family. They were quite the amusing pair!

Of course, Brady and Austin both had their superheroes as kids. I can still see Brady dressed up in his Batman costume, standing on my dining room chair to reach the mirror and look at himself. What precious memories! They both had Power Rangers suits and Spiderman costumes. You name it, they were into it. Seems that each Christmas was a different "theme," which made it sort of easy for us grandparents, once we knew what it was. The same way with their birthdays. Star Wars is still very much a part of Brady's interests because this past Christmas, I know he received some Star Wars gifts that made him extremely happy. Ha ha. And him a pastor! By the way, Brady is also the father of a wonderful boy named Beau Andrew Howard, born on April 3, 2015. He and Savannah are also the proud parents of a little daughter named Adeline Grace who was born on August 31, 2017.

Of course, when A and B were small, we had our little cowboys *for sure*! They loved watching the cowboys and Indians on TV with Poppy, Paw Paw, and their dad. I guess all men, old or young, love the Western Channel on TV. They had their different types of entertainment at both sets of grandparents. But you could be sure of one thing—whichever house they were visiting, they were the absolute center of attention while they were there. Were they spoiled? Nah! Never happened! It was the real delight for Granny Sweet Pea and me

THE MAKING OF A WONDERFUL LIFE

to be actively involved as babysitters for those boys much of the time as they were growing up. How swiftly that time has passed!

I will never forget the modern-looking bright green and yellow plastic convertible car Austin loved so much. He would drive it all around in our apartment. He was a great mechanic and had his own tools (and any of Poppy's he could get his hands on!). He would work so hard repairing his car every time he drove it. He was very meticulous at keeping it nice and clean, too. In the summer months, he would take it outside and wash it on our little back deck. Such great memories I have of seeing that little blond-haired blue-eyed boy working hour after hour on his green machine.

When Brady was little, he liked to entertain us by playing his musical instruments. Austin liked to work. Now Brady is in the ministry, preaching, teaching, and singing, and Austin is in college but working every spare moment of his life either with their cattle farm or on construction sites. However, God has also gifted him musically as well, and he can sing and play and make a great addition to our worship and praise band at church each Sunday morning. He actually has come into his own as a worship leader. I'm so thankful for both of these grandsons and the gifts they are using for the Lord.

I prayed for my grandchildren from the time they were born, actually even before they were born, that God would put a hedge of protection around them and keep them from the wiles of the devil and direct their paths in the right way. I know I was always the hypercritical grammy when it came to some of the TV shows that they would watch. There seemed to be such hidden agendas in some of the cartoons that I felt like they were just sending subliminal messages and actually brainwashing our little ones.

It was so much fun for us to watch the boys play "make believe" and imagining they were a part of Poppy and Uncle Buddy's gospel singing group and traveling band. In fact, I can remember Brady doing that when he was just a baby boy, two or three years old. He would play on our stairway when we were living in a duplex apartment on Sentry Oak Court. He loved to pretend that the stairs were Poppy and Buddy's big Silver Eagle bus, and he was a part of their band. He'd load his guitars and all sorts of little carrying cases onto his bus. He was hauling his "equipment." I'd fix him a broom handle with a paper plate on the end of it for his steering wheel, and he would sit on the second step of the stairwell and go on long "trips" to sing the gospel all over America. We had a cute little boy next door to us in the duplex, and he would come over and bring his toy guitar, too. Poppy and I would sometimes make ourselves something to play, like drums or washboards, and we would have us quite the traveling band!

It seems like only yesterday, those boys were just little fellas, and now Brady is twenty-nine and married to Savannah, and Austin is twenty-five and married to Savannah's sister, Suzanne. "Where has the time gone?" Now we start a new cycle with those Howard boys and their little ones. They'll grow up as double cousins. How neat is that?

Albania: The Next Step

After Roger came back from his first trip to Albania in March 1994, and we totally surrendered to this new ministry of working with Hope for the World in providing much-needed funds for the Albanian orphans, we had to seek the Lord's leading as to the best way to go about this monumental task.

We had taken about four years away from our prior life of evangelism as a family while Roger devoted all of his time to the gospel music industry and getting Buddy established in his career. "Mullins & Co.," Buddy's band, was signed by a booking agency in Nashville, secured a record contract, and stayed pretty busy in the field of Christian music. We had assisted with the management side of their musical career for a while, but now it was time for us to let go of those reins and concentrate on the new ministry God had called us to—helping orphans in one of the poorest countries of Eastern Europe, Albania. They were now our newest love!

Just how were we going to raise our own personal support along with funds to supply the needs of these precious orphan children in Albania? Only God knew. It was our job to accept the assignment and trust in him fully. It was his job to provide what we needed.

Hope for the World was already set up as a nonprofit organization in America. Roger had a number of initial meetings with the board of directors of Hope for the World and even became a member of that board himself about as soon as he surrendered to the calling. He and I prayed and asked God not only to lead us and direct us in the right paths in securing our own personal support as full-time missionaries but also to show us ways and methods of raising the needed funds to provide for the orphans. At that time, our commitment in Albania was to one large orphanage in the capital city of Tirana, plus a guesthouse that Hope for the World also owned in the city.

This guesthouse was not very large, with rooms furnished with bunk beds. Men shared one room, and ladies shared the other. Also, an apartment was available upstairs for some of the American workers who were living in Albania and working with Hope for the World. The guesthouse provided free lodging and meals for various guests who visited Albania to assist in the ministry. Also in-country missionaries who came from distant villages and towns to stay in Tirana for a day or so to conduct business would often stay at the guesthouse. There was a very nominal fee for room and board for those guests. We had a wonderful cook on the premises named Like (pronounced "Lee-kah") Hafizi. Her husband, Memtaz, was the government director of the Tirana school-age orphanage. She could fix some of the best food, and it was always prepared with much love and care as she truly appreciated the American missionaries who had come to help their country. We immediately came to love her as a sister, even though we did not speak her language nor she ours. Thank the Lord for some good interpreters. They were not always available, however, and this was when I would really try to learn the language when I "had to!" I love the challenge of a foreign language, so from the beginning I have tried to learn enough phrases and words to be able to at least greet the people in their native tongue. They love that!

We had assembled a small staff of an Albanian family who were mainly serving in the guesthouse as maid, driver, and guard at that time. They had small salaries from Hope for the World, but it was still much more than they could possibly earn in their own country. At the time we began our work there, the unemployment rate was about 75 percent, and the average wage was equal to $25 per *month*! Our Albanian employees were very committed to their jobs since they depended on these funds that came from Hope for the World each month. All the American missionaries or volunteer workers were self-funded or had raised their own personal support as missionaries.

After we had been in the country for a while, Roger realized what a real financial burden the guesthouse was for Hope for the

World and decided it was best to close it. Sadly, he had to tell those Albanian employees that he was going to close the guesthouse, which meant their jobs would go, too. When Roger met with the Albanians to give them the news, he had a friend from America with him at the meeting. That ended up being a good thing since the Albanian man actually came after Roger physically and was going to beat him up. It was a little rough for a while, but they pulled him back and Roger was not hurt. A positive thing that resulted concerning the guesthouse was that we were able to "give" it over to another Christian NGO from Holland, and they were happy to have it. I don't recall if those Albanian employees continued with that organization or not. This was a financial load off the budget that had been put in place before we came on board.

There had also been other commitments made with the government in contract form for aid to the orphanage, so the monthly budget at the outset of our ministry with Hope for the World was approximately $3,000 per month. That seemed like a huge amount for Roger and me to raise, but we knew it would happen if God was in it. We also had to begin raising our own support as well. Fortunately, we had a small group of monthly supporters when we were in evangelism. We called them "Torchbearers." They made monthly donations to our own 501(c)(3) corporation known as "Roger Mullins Evangelistic Association, Inc." during the years we lived on the road in a bus. These Torchbearers' donations supplemented our income at that time due to the heavy expenses connected with living on the road and keeping our bus repaired, fueled, and rolling. Love offerings were a blessing, but because we did not set any price at all for our ministry, and would not turn down even the smallest of churches for meetings, there were many times that there was a lot more "love" than "offering," and it was difficult to make ends meet, to say the least. That is what necessitated us having the Torchbearers as a monthly support group.

We had also suspended our monthly newsletter for about four years, but we immediately started it back into circulation. We did not pick up all of the addresses we had, and we had no way of knowing which ones would still be accurate until we sent out our first letters. We began writing a monthly newsletter once again and letting people know about this transition we had made into missions. We were blessed to hear from some of our dear friends and former "Torchbearers," and some were interested in becoming a help in this mission work. What a joy that was to us.

One of those families was Carl and Vernice Howard out in San Antonio, Texas, along with their two sons and one daughter. If you have read my book subtitled *Joyous Journey*, you have already been introduced to this family. They immediately jumped right in and began not only supporting us personally but also taking a vital role in providing some of the much-needed monthly funding for the orphans. They have been true partners with us through the years in this ministry, and we know God placed them in our path in the 1980s, and they are still with us today, though we are all getting "old." Ha ha. Vernice isn't! (She's the only one!)

Roger also began to call some of his pastor friends all around the country where we had held revivals. Some of them were very welcoming to our transition and were interested in having us come to their church to present this Albanian orphan ministry. However, many of them had totally lost interest in us and our ministry when Roger had taken the four-year stint in gospel music to get Buddy established. So gaining supporting churches and raising sufficient monthly support for our family were not an easy task. Also, some pastors didn't understand the concept that we would be missionaries but would be living in America and not in Albania. They didn't seem to grasp the idea that someone had to work on *this* side of the world in order to provide funding for all that was happening on that other side of the world.

There were other churches we were acquainted with who were not interested in any mission work that was not primarily planting churches, even though Hope for the World was among the very first Christian organizations to plant churches in Albania which are all still standing and flourishing to this day. It just was not "our calling" to plant a church but to plant the seed of the Gospel in the hearts of boys and girls. So you can imagine that it was not an easy road, getting our new ministry up and rolling and self-supporting.

Thankfully, we did begin to get invited to many churches asking us to come and tell them about the country of Albania and our new ministry that God had laid so heavily on our hearts. We would go and share the stories of the Albanian orphans and their dire needs.

Our first slide show was from one of the early American missionaries, Dave Young. Dave went in as a layman and led so many to Christ he had to come back to America, be ordained, and go back and start New Hope Baptist Church in Tirana where many of our own staff members are members to this day. Brother Dave and Sister Faye Young gave their very best years and physical strength to the work there in Tirana. We were blessed to be able to minister with them out in the villages as well as in their beautiful church that began upstairs over a pool hall in the early days. As a matter of fact, our president, Perparim Demcellari, and his family were led to Christ by Brother David, and he also led Perparim through a full Bible college curriculum which led to him also becoming an ordained minister. Brother Dave Young loaned us his slides, as I mentioned, and we made up a presentation to show from church to church. The pictures literally would speak to the hearts of Christian people everywhere, and God began to build his work and our ministry in Albania to the orphans. In this way, we began to pick up a support base. It was very different for Roger and me to be going out all by ourselves, when we had always had the whole family or a group of young men with us to present a full music program, but we learned a few duets to sing together, and I'd throw in a piano solo or two. Roger has always had a great repertoire of solos to sing plus his humorous songs and stories that always endeared people to him. So we went out and did what we could, and God was faithful to provide our needs over and over again.

No church was more helpful and encouraging to us than our own home church, Glen Haven Baptist. At that time, the church was located in Decatur, Georgia. Glen Haven immediately put us on their list as full-time missionaries and began to support us monthly. They continue to support our ministry to this day. Not only that, they were some of the very first to give special love offerings for many of the urgent needs in Albania for the orphanage. Pastor Ralph Easterwood was the senior pastor at that time, and he had a huge heart for missions and a real gift at raising funds for many, many worldwide ministries. He was always open to our ministry and to any of our people from Albania or other American missionaries who worked with us in that country. Glen Haven has always been a tremendously mission-minded church, and I believe that is one of the reasons they have been so blessed through the years. We realize that we probably would not still be in this work if it was not for this wonderful "home base." When Pastor Ralph retired at age seventy-five, his assistant pastor, Stan Berrong, became the senior pastor. Under his leadership, our church continues to be a huge part of the work of Hope for the World in Albania. Glen Haven, now located in McDonough, Georgia, has recently built a new and very beautiful sanctuary and office complex, and the congregation has grown remarkably over the past several years. We thank the Lord for their heart for our ministry and for their visits to see the work in Albania.

So many Glen Haven members are sponsors of our orphan children in Albania. Many other members of our home church, along with some very wonderful supporters we have had behind us for years as a result of our monthly newsletter, helped us to completely furnish the Hope Center for Teens when it was opened in 2010. It is a great blessing to belong to a body of believers like we have had at Glen Haven since we moved to Georgia in 1990.

Roger worked tirelessly, through phone calls and getting into churches, to present our ministry. I put in many hours in our office, rebuilding a mailing list and writing monthly newsletters. We also started a sponsorship program for the orphans where people could choose an orphan to sponsor and contribute monthly to their needs through Hope for the World. This helped us raise our monthly budget each month and provided for the work we were doing in Albania for these children and also paid the small salaries of our Albanian staff. When I say "small salaries," I want you to know that their monthly salaries would not even begin to equal many *weekly* wages of people here in America. Yet they each work tirelessly every single day, usually six days a week.

It just seems that whenever God would open the door in Albania and we would accept the invitation of the Albanian government to help one more orphanage in that country, God would give us the peace to step further out by faith. He would grow our group of supporting churches, sponsors, or individual supporters to meet that need. Now mind you, in all of the years we have been in this work, we never have had what you would call a "slush fund" sitting here in the office. The funds simply come in month by month, just in time to meet the budget as it has continued to grow through the years.

However, we want to give God all of the praise as it is truly amazing for us to see how he has provided for the needs of this work since its inception. He was doing it then, and he continues to do it to this day. We try to stay in step with him, be obedient servants, and stay willing to be used to reach this group of people in Albania for his glory. We are so very appreciative of those who actually read and respond so well to the needs as we present them in our monthly newsletter. We learned a scripture in the Bible a long time ago that has been very important in this ministry. It says in James 4:2: "Ye have not because ye ask not." We have learned through the years that people need to "know the need" in order to respond to that need.

I would love to be able to tell you that my sweet husband doesn't sweat it out from month to month and pray and worry some (sometimes a lot) about whether or not the budget is going to come in that month. However, I cannot tell you that. He definitely feels the weight of this responsibility constantly. It never leaves his mind. In fact, during the first years of the ministry, it showed up on him with an ulcerated stomach. I am happy to say, however, that through the years, as we have seen God continue to supply over and over again, his ulcers improved, and he really doesn't deal with them anymore.

I honestly don't know how Roger has carried all of the stress of the financial commitments we have in Albania through these twenty plus years. It's easy to say, "Just trust the Lord," but it's not always easy to do. Fear and doubt and discouragement are big attacks of the enemy. I just know that I have always tried to be Roger's encourager when it comes to God's faithfulness. He has certainly had to pray daily as he makes his trip to the post office, which he has dubbed his "wailing wall." This is where the funds come in each month, mostly through the mail. When it seems we are not going to make it some month, I usually go into his office and just remind him that God has not missed a month yet. Can we expect him to cop out on us this month? We take it to the Lord in prayer. We realize that his ways are not our ways, and his ways are past finding out sometimes right until the very last minute. But praise the Lord! I'm so happy to relate in this book that he has seen us through some really awesome needs and primarily a current monthly budget of $25,000 each month. We are so blessed to be a part of this ministry, and we could not figure out how God plans to handle these needs in any given month, we just know that he *does*!

It is a difficult thing to be 100 percent wrapped up in a ministry to which God has called you, and to which you have given so many years of your life, and not think of it as "*my* ministry." In actual truth, it's "God's ministry." I think if there is one thing we battle as missionaries, it is that truth, especially when we were in on the very birth stages of the ministry and feel a personal responsibility to do all we can to keep it going. We almost think that without "us," it would not be there, which of course is not true. We see the very best growth and realization of visions on the field, when we take our hands off and quit trying and start trusting! So hard to do! Easy to say and makes for some good preaching! Lord help us to let go and let God!

In our heart of hearts, we truly believe that this work in Albania that was begun in the early 1990s is 100 percent God's ministry. We feel greatly honored and privileged to just be in on it. We get weary at times, yes, but we are so excited at the many, many wonderful blessings of God that have transpired through the years. We would not have wanted him to have chosen anyone else to work in this particular vineyard. It has been, and continues to be, an awesome experience that we would not trade for any other in this lifetime.

In the beginning stages, we were helping provide the essentials of life for orphans in the school-age orphanage in Tirana, Albania. There were about one hundred seventy children in that home at the time. We were also trying to provide some funds to help a special deaf orphanage in the city as well. Our contract was with the Ministries of Labor and Social Services in the country. Knowing that this would be part of Roger's role in Albania was really a little scary to me. Meeting with government officials? Wow! My man was starting to walk in some really high cotton! I was so proud of him, also a little worried too, but that just meant we had more for which to trust God. Seems like every day we were beginning to walk on new paths in this life. It has been quite a faith journey now that I look back on it and try to explain it.

Cherie's First Trip to Albania

I remember how thrilled I was with the fact that Roger was going back and forth to Albania and coming in telling me about all of the experiences he had while there and the many different people he had met. He didn't share too much with me about the culture, the food, and the things women like to know, because to be honest, they were not things that captured his attention. He was on a mission to help the suffering orphan children, and mainly he was meeting with the Albanian director, Memtaz Hafizi, with the Americans who were there working with the kids and with some other American pastors who were there as missionaries and planting churches in Albania. Roger's time and thoughts were mainly involved with these people.

That being said, when I went with him in 1995 for my very first time, there was a lot that I saw with my own eyes and experienced in my heart and spirit that was totally new. The traveling in itself was quite an experience as we could never just fly from Atlanta to Albania. No airlines were making that connection. And they still do not fly directly from America to Albania. There is always a layover or connecting flight somewhere in Europe, and usually somewhere else in the United States, before going to Europe. I recall that the first flights we were taking were on Swissair that flew out of Atlanta, and if I remember correctly, they flew right to Zurich where we would get our connecting flight to Tirana, Albania.

It was fun flying on Swissair and listening to all of the announcements from the cockpit and from the flight attendants in both German and in English. They were very nice planes and wonderful crews. The food was always delicious, too, and that's a lot to say about airplane food. You could tell that they took pride in serving some products and dishes that were definitely Swiss based. There were many different types of cheese, for instance. Each time our tray was served, you could count on at least two different cheeses with our meal. And bread in abundance, too! They would often pass through the aisles with baskets of extra rolls during and after the course of the meal. And those chocolates! Oh, my goodness! Swiss chocolates! Nothing like them!

At the Zurich airport, I began doing something that has since become sort of a "signature" for me. While awaiting our connecting flight, I would always have time to wander through the shops. There were so many things there to buy, but many were way too expensive, and I could not pack or carry them very easily. And then I found a little shop that sold all handmade items, and a lot of them were handkerchiefs, etc. It was there that I began my collection of colorful bandana-like handkerchiefs. The ones I bought in Switzerland always had either the Swiss cow with a cowbell around its neck or their national symbol, Edelweiss, a flower that grows high up in the Alps. I saw these colorful hankies as both practical, decorative, and a souvenir from Switzerland, so this is what I began to buy for myself. It took up absolutely no room in my luggage or my purse and weighed nearly nothing and had many practical uses. I use them for a decorative accessory out of a pocket of my purse, a bib to keep me from dropping food onto myself when eating in my best clothing, a shield from Roger's spray when we are singing duets, and even as a real handkerchief at times. There is no end to the uses, but I'll spare you.

I did manage to buy some Swiss chocolates as gifts to bring home to family and close friends. One time, I bought a cute Swiss hat for my very first grandson, Brady. Things of that nature were usually very pricey, however. We were always on a lookout for a Coke bottle for Brother Ralph (our pastor at that time) as he was a collector of unusual Coca-Cola bottles. We tried to bring one from any different country we traveled through if at all possible. Brother Eddie Weik, another friend and brother in our church, always asked us to bring him a rock from each country. His rock collection is really quite amazing!

Since we were traveling through Zurich and flying Swissair so much of the time, we later decided that we would add a special little side trip to Lucerne, Switzerland, on the way back home and do some sightseeing in Switzerland. Oh, I so loved that! We did that on two or three different trips with various friends. Switzerland is so beautiful especially in the rural areas where the farmland is so meticulously laid out and the cows actually do graze along the meadowlands and up the mountainsides, proudly ringing their cowbells, playing their own music as they graze.

I will never forget going through the little shops in Lucerne. There were so many colorful things to buy. I mainly went into the "tourist traps," as that is where I could find something I thought I could afford. One time, however, Roger let me go into a clock shop, and we actually bought our very first (and only) cuckoo clock made right there in Switzerland. It had the yodelers on it that would come out and yodel every hour, and the pretty music box would play and they would dance every half hour. I loved my clock, and I was very faithful to wind it by pulling the weights at least twice a day to keep it running and functioning for a long, long time.

Now let me get back on track and tell you about my first time entering Albania. I can remember sitting by a window in the plane as we flew into the country. The flight from Zurich to Tirana is approximately two hours. As we approached Tirana, the capital city of Albania, I remember looking for skyscrapers, but there were none in view. In fact, as I looked down, it looked more like I was looking at something similar to chicken houses since the first buildings I saw were one story and very old looking. When I saw the airport, it was also very small, one story, and not very impressive to say the least.

When we landed, they sent a big bus out onto the airstrip or tarmac to load us up and take us into the little airport. The bus was nearly as big as the facility itself. When we got inside, we were all handed a form to fill out (wherever we could find a place to prop up and write on it). This was to give them explicit information as to where we would be staying while there. It was to tell them how many nights and days we would be there and the nature of our visit. There were no tables, shelves, or anything of that type for us to write on, only a very tiny ledge alongside the customs windows. We had to stand in line and be cleared by a customs official and then directed to another area where we each had to pay an entry fee of ten dollars as we came into Albania. (This fee has since been discontinued.)

Of course, most women are always looking for the nearest restroom, and I was no exception. Wouldn't you know, there was not one to be had in this particular side of the airport! They just had one for departing flights, none for arrivals. There also was no such thing as a luggage carousel for our bags to arrive on. We just went to another section of the little airport where people were bunched up as close as they could get to the outside door while baggage was literally being thrown inside the building by the baggage handlers. There was no order or procedure really; it was up to us to elbow our way into the middle of the crowd and wait and watch for our own pieces and then try to squeeze our way through to claim them.

Roger had been there before, so he knew the ropes, and I just stayed back and waited for him and watched and listened to this strange Albanian language called Shqip. You pronounce that word just like it was "Ship," well, nearly anyway. If you want to know the truth, since I have been there all these years and have learned a lot of the language and the sounds of their alphabet, it is really pronounced as if it were spelled S-H-C-H-I-P. Hard to say? It really is! But that's the way they say it. The "q" has the sound of "ch." Oh, to speak this language is difficult! But I loved listening to it and wondering what they were saying as we were arriving. I definitely could understand when they would say "Ahme-reek" or "Ahmeri-kahn." That was us!

I soon saw that Roger had made a very special friend there in the baggage area of the airport. I wish I could remember her name. I can still see her in my mind's eye. She was a short stocky Albanian woman who was very strong and made her presence known as far as being a help to us in collecting all of our bags. Of course, she was working for tips, and Roger had already registered in her mind as a "good" tipper, so when she saw us arrive, she began immediately to follow him around as he pointed to our luggage. It seemed strange to me for him to let this woman tote our bags and pile them onto a baggage carrier, but that was the custom, and it was her job, so we stood back and watched her work. She smiled at me, and I tried to greet her with my one little greeting word that I knew that stood for "good morning" or "good afternoon." I had learned those words because I do like to at least appear to be friendly when visiting another country.

Our party that was awaiting us was not allowed to come into the airport. They had to wait outside, and so when we would finally get all the baggage and clear the customs camera with our luggage (if it was working that day), we were free to go out and meet them. I can remember being met by some of the American people with Hope for the World, along with some Albanians as well. They had a van and loaded everything into the back of the van, and we all got inside and away we went, as quickly as we could. I still had not found a ladies' restroom by the way. I had let Roger know, and he let them know, so they were going to accommodate me as soon as possible, but there was really nothing on our way where they could stop for me. We had about an hour or more drive to get to the Hope for the World guesthouse. I just know it seemed like a very long ride, and I was in total discomfort.

I remember how extremely rough the roads were everywhere. They were all dirt roads with huge potholes. You couldn't travel fast at all. Also, there were mud puddles everywhere from the rain. You didn't see very many vehicles on the road at that time. More horse-drawn carts with sometimes just two people riding and other times whole families. They were loaded with all sorts of goods and hay bales, etc. It was really something to see! I was truly fascinated by these horse-drawn carts and already had an urge to ride on one of them before leaving the country. Our American missionaries, Hugh and Debbie Hoffman, heard my wish and made sure one day before I left Albania that they hailed a wagon with two young boys in it and asked them if I could ride. They obliged, and I had the ride of my life that day! Certainly an experience to remember. And a sight to see, I'm sure.

The guesthouse was on a muddy street, but even so, the yard around the house was walled by concrete and had a big iron gate that stayed locked. On top of the walls everywhere, you would see what looked like steel picket fencing. Sharp points and glass shards on top of each rod. This, we were told, was part of their defense system under communism. They had been told by their dictator that the Americans would be jumping out of planes and coming to attack them. These sharp fences were to pierce and injure the invaders. It was really very sad to see this all over the country wherever we would go. The streets were lined by these walls and armored fences on top of them.

No matter how small the yard around a house, it would always be enclosed, and gated, and a guard posted on the property to allow or not allow vehicles access. This was so foreign to me and so depressing. Living in the "Land of the Free" automatically began to mean more to me than ever before. The guard at the gate was happy to welcome us from America! He, of course, spoke no English at all, but he knew that we were with Hope for the World, the owners of the guesthouse and, hence, his employer. That brought a smile from him as soon as we arrived. All the money he received in the world came to him from our organization. I might say right here that what we had to pay employees at that time was so very miniscule as they had all been living on $25 per month under communism. So you can see that even if we doubled their pay, it was not much money according to American standards, but it was way more than they were used to receiving.

At the guesthouse, we had our wonderful cook as I mentioned earlier on. Her name was Like (pronounced Leekah), and she was married to the director of the school-age orphanage in the capital city. His name was Memtaz. I immediately bonded with this woman. She was a great cook and prepared foods that Americans could enjoy very much. She had a very fun personality, and we got along marvelously. Some of our full-time American missionaries had coached her on some special recipes, I feel sure, and we did not lack for good food while we were there as her guests for meals. Memtaz became an instant good friend of Roger's, and as he did not have much longer to work for the Albanian government before he would have to retire, Roger saw fit to hire him as a staff director for Hope for the World in Albania. Memtaz had been saved under the leadership of Hope for the World missionaries and was a new Christian, and it was very refreshing to see his love for the children and his heart to help in all the ways he could.

Let me pause here and insert some information concerning Memtaz Hafizi. We had some wonderful years working with Memtaz. We were blessed to bring him to our home in Georgia for a visit one time. I will never forget how he loved to sit on my front porch in the rocker and just enjoy the wooded area around my house. He said he really loved how "green" Georgia was. We are so happy he got to come here. (He actually was accompanying his daughter, Vera, who was a high school graduate and had won the lottery in her country to be able to come to America for employment. She had met some American missionaries from Grand Rapids, Michigan, who had been to Albania working with Hope for the World. They made it possible for her to have a home with them, and she was employed by Radio Bible Class in Grand Rapids, Michigan, where she met her husband.) During Memtaz and Vera's visit, we had to buy clothing for both of them as their luggage got lost, and they never got it back!

When we bought Memtaz's clothes, he wanted them to be like Roger's. If we took him out to eat, he wanted to order whatever Roger ordered on the menu. It was just so much fun having him here. Of course, we had to have an interpreter with him which was also fun, and there was an Albanian who was a great interpreter and lived not far away in Alabama, so he came to stay with us while we had our guests from Albania. We spoke absolutely no Albanian in those days, and they spoke no English. We had Memtaz as our Albanian director until the year 1999 when he became very ill with cancer. They had no way to treat it in Albania and, sometimes, no way of actually diagnosing it early enough for any kind of treatment back then. Our hearts broke when we learned that he had become critically ill in Albania, and in a very short time, his life on earth was over from this illness.

We loved his widow, Like, and decided then and there that we would continue taking care of her financially by giving her Memtaz's salary each month, which we did until she later was able to move to America with her daughter, Vera, who was able to provide for her. Vera's story is another wonderful blessing from God that we saw happen. She was a very sweet and very intelligent young Albanian girl and had been given an opportunity to come to America and live with that family in Michigan who had been doing mission work in Albania. She moved to the Grand Rapids area and was able to get work for the Radio Bible Class ministry there. She met a Baptist pastor's son, Steve Harrison, and they fell in love and married. They have a wonderful Christian home and children who are growing up not only physically but spiritually. Vera was able to get her mother, Like, over to Michigan from Albania to live with them.

Vera's brother, Redi, is also in America with his family as well as other family members who have been able to emigrate to the United States through the years. They love God and America with their whole hearts, and they keep in touch with us pretty regularly. It is such a blessing to see how these lives were touched by the Lord under the missionaries working with Hope for the World in Albania and how they continue to "grow and glow" for the Lord. Many Albanian families have come to America now through so many different ways. Some through marriage, some through adoption, some through college opportunities, but all because of the spread of the Gospel through missionaries.

One of the things I distinctly remember seeing that was a bit disturbing to me was the way people transported their loaves of bread from the local bakeries. It appeared that they must not have had any grocery bags of any type at that time, at least not at the bakery, so men and women could be seen riding their bicycles down the street with a baked loaf of bread, with no wrapper of any kind, under their arm. It did not seem to be customary to keep the bread in any type of enclosure either once it had been sliced for meals. I did not ever see anything like our ziplock bags in which to store things to keep them fresh. The bread would just sit out and get harder and harder between meals. I learned that bread was a huge staple of the average citizen's diet. That and a huge block of white cheese, goat cheese I believe it was, as they raised a lot of goats in Albania and not too many cows.

I'll never forget going to the cheese store with Debbie Hoffman who was on our staff. There was so much cheese stacked up on those counters in huge chunks and rounds. Wow! I mean like five-foot-tall stacks of round white cheese. Each round about a foot thick! I'll never forget it. I asked them if it was OK for me to take pictures, and they were so kind and let me take all the photos I wanted. It was very obvious that they were used to selling lots of this cheese. I soon learned that this was one of the food staples in each home.

Debbie took me that day to the huge open market. Vegetables and fruits were not a surprise to me, except for the fact that they were large and beautiful and organically grown and so inexpensive! There were also olives everywhere in huge baskets, oh my goodness! So many different varieties! I wasn't sure if all of these things were grown in Albania, but I sort of thought at that time they possibly were brought in from Greece or other neighboring countries. I could have been dead wrong, but that was what I thought at the time since Albania was such a poverty-stricken country back then. The meat market was a place that I could not linger as there were many sheep and goats and some other animals hanging there, entire carcasses, stripped of their hide only.

It was in Albania that I first began to dip my bread into olive oil, sort of sopping it, much as we do now in the nice Italian restaurants here in America. It took a little getting used to that, and their oil was not as refined as our "extra virgin" olive oil here. It seemed to be a little thicker. Now as far as olives are concerned, I absolutely love olives, and we had olives every single meal! Those, along with the cheese, which was much like feta cheese, seemed to appear as side dishes along with every meal we enjoyed while there. Yogurt was another main dish. They made a sort of dip that went on the table with fresh vegetables like tomatoes and cucumbers. I'm not sure how it was made, but I could taste some cucumbers and onions very finely chopped and mixed in this yogurt, and I learned to love it. Their country is blessed with olive trees, and it is one of their main sources of income, both the fruit and the oil. I will say this about that Albanian olive oil, it certainly kept your insides well lubricated and made for no digestive problems if you know what I mean. Ha ha!

One of my favorite things to eat in Albania was the soups that were made by our Albanian cook. They were very tasty and mainly made from vegetables in a creamy broth. You couldn't really tell what vegetables were in the soups because they were pureed. I love soup, and they would have it nearly every meal as our first course. Breakfast would consist of boiled eggs, various cheeses, olives, bread, and sometimes some fruit preserves to spread on the bread. I believe some of them also ate a type of fish for breakfast. I have never been, and am not today, a fish-eater. I don't recall ever having a piece of bacon or having my bread toasted in Albania, not back in those early days anyhow. That is all changing now in more recent years.

There were different types of rooms at the guesthouse, but most of them had bunk beds, and they would sleep either a whole family, a group of men, or a group of women in the same room. I do recall, however, that on our first visit, they let Roger and me have a private room with a king-sized bed. It may have belonged to the Hoffmans, the American couple who were part of the Hope for the World staff from the very beginning. I really cannot remember why we rated such a big bed. We found that bed to be extremely hard! They do not use box springs, just an actual box (wooden) under a thin mattress. Our mattress was a little thicker than most of the others, but even the mattresses are very, very firm and are just laid on boards as a foundation. It is pretty hard for people who have hip issues or sciatic nerve problems, or arthritis, all of which I have had through the years. But on the other hand, it may be that this type of bed was what I needed to sleep on at home to keep me from having any of those problems. I remember that while we were there, we got so tired each day that by bedtime I don't think it really mattered what I laid on; I was going to sleep, that's for sure! They could probably have hung us on a hook, and we would have slept!

At that time, there was a young couple working there at the guesthouse. I do not recall their names, but the lady helped Like with some of the cooking and serving and also did chambermaid work. Her husband would handle things such as driving the vehicle for our organization, guarding the gate, maintaining the property, etc. There was an older man there, too, whose job was to open and close the gate when someone arrived or departed. This man was probably not as old as he looked. We soon learned that no one in Albania was usually as old as they looked. They looked old because the oppression they suffered under communism truly showed in their faces and their bodies as well. That was something we readily noticed.

    I will never forget watching the street sweepers everywhere we would travel, sweeping the streets in front of buildings with their homemade brooms. These ladies wore very long skirts and layers of clothing, and on their heads would be a scarf, or what I had always called a babushka, to keep the dirt out of their hair as they swept the torn-up sidewalks. There was truly not a smooth street or sidewalk anywhere in the country at that time. Many places looked like they had been bombed or an earthquake had come and heaved up the concrete. I can remember trying to walk down the sidewalks along the busy streets and coming upon a deep hole in the pavement where chunks of concrete were simply gone. There was never any type of caution sign or safety fence around any of these holes. I think this is when I began to realize that we in America take so many things for granted, and I was truly in a third-world country which was the poorest in Eastern Europe at that time. My heart ached for the Albanian people and their country.

    Our work in Albania at that particular time was pretty well centered around the orphanage in Tirana and the guesthouse. We did not have to take any lengthy drives at first to the city of Shkodra. That began a year or so after we started coming to Albania. It was a good thing, because the roads around the city were nothing but one deep rut and pothole after another. When it rained, these potholes were full of water, of course, and nearly impassable.

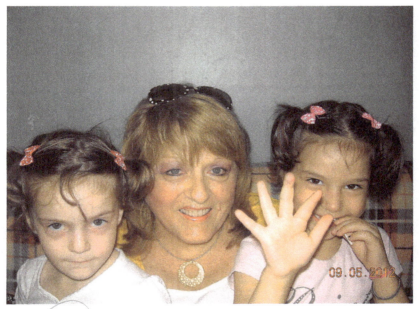

Cherie with a couple of the little ones from the orphanage

Tirana Orphanage

I remember well my very first visit to the orphanage in Tirana. Oh my goodness, it was so very, very pitiful. It was a large block building, about four stories tall with huge windows that opened out with a crank handle. The sad thing was that most of the windows were broken out, and the crank handles didn't work either, so you may as well say there were "no windows." Even if they had one or two windows that worked, they were usually thrown wide open, and this was not summer weather either. I soon figured out that part of the reason for being open all the time was due to the stench inside the building because of the very unsanitary conditions and the many children who were regular bed wetters. There was also insufficient laundry equipment to keep up with clothing, let alone, for washing the bedding. It was cold, and rainy, and not at all warm anywhere in that building. It was nearly like living outside.

The children played on the balconies or climbed from window to window on ledges that were not very wide or safe at all. It absolutely scared me to death to see how they were like little monkeys crawling all around. There was little or no electricity or lights in the building. Then I learned that they only had electricity within the city for a very few hours every day. It did make that building very dark. It was also very clammy, cold, dirty, and loud. Of course, that was to be expected with the large number of children running through the hallways, the sound echoing off the high ceilings, block walls, etc. We were on tour with the government director, Memtaz (Like's husband). He was a kind, sweet-natured, and rather soft-spoken gentleman. We, of course, had to use an interpreter as he spoke no English and we, of course, did not speak Shqip. So he graciously showed us all over the building, giving us our first glimpse of some of the worst living conditions you could ever imagine for a human being.

The cots that the children were sleeping on had such sunken mattresses that they almost looked like hammocks on the frames of the metal beds. It broke my heart. As I said earlier, the stench of urine was very predominant in the rooms where the smallest children slept. My heart hurt so for those children. I wanted to go and buy all of them brand new beds and mattresses and new warm blankets with nice fluffy pillows. There were none in Albania to be bought, however. I made that a personal project when I came home from Albania. We were able to buy new mattresses, pillows, and blankets for them within a short time. I can remember packing boxes filled with pillows and sending them over on the military planes we were blessed to have at our disposal through the US government's "Denton Amendment." It took a little longer to get new beds, but I will never forget when we went back to Albania and saw that the children were sleeping in wooden bunk beds instead of those rusty iron cots and that they all had nice warm blankets and pillows for the first time. This is true of all of the orphanages we worked with in Albania through the years. Their sleeping conditions were not only uncomfortable, but also their orphanages were very, very cold during the winter months. When we walked through the rooms where the little ones were asleep for their naps during the daytime, we could see their breath; it was so cold.

There were over 170 children in the Zyber Hallulli Orphanage in Tirana. They had huge sleeping barracks, girls in one room, guys in the other. Each floor was for different ages of children. The older ones were higher up in the building, but their accommodations were not much, if any, better. They just didn't wet their beds, so that was at least an improvement in the odor.

As we went into the teenage girls' barracks in that building, we were taken outside of their rooms onto their balcony that had a short wall with a wide ledge. On these ledges were basins for the girls to wash their own things and especially certain items they had to use instead of feminine hygiene products like we have for girls.

They had no feminine products like that in Albania, at least none for the orphans. I'm not sure if they even had them for the women in general. They had to use old rags, and each girl had to wash those rags and take care of their monthly needs in that way. Can you imagine? My heart just continued to break, and I wept for these girls as I walked around the area. I determined right then that we needed to put feminine hygiene products at the very top of the list and somehow see that these girls had things they needed on a regular basis. And we did, praise the Lord! In looking at all of the conditions there, it was very hard to know where to start first in the order of helping, providing, and improving life for them.

We wanted to love them to Jesus, and the best way was to care enough for them to provide the very essentials of life and make things easier for them. When you do that, then they pose the question, "Why do you do these things for us?" "Why do you come from America all the way over here and spend your money to help us?" "Why don't you just live and be happy in your own country and not worry about us?" We were asked these questions many times by the children. They could not figure out why we were there and why we wanted to help them.

It was through loving them and supplying them with food, clothing, bedding, and even a furnace to heat their huge building that we would get to tell them about the one who loved us so much he gave his only begotten Son for us. He loved us so much he left heaven's perfection and came to a lowly manger and was born in the humblest manner to show us that he truly cared for us and loved us. We would tell them we were trying to follow his example. There are so many great opportunities to share Christ through humanitarian efforts. No one really knows until you have been there and done that. You don't have to be a missionary to any foreign country; we can do it right here in America if we will just open our eyes and hearts and look around us.

This made me think of a neat illustration my daughter, Cindy, brought to me from a visit she made to her optometrist. She was trying to convert from regular glasses to the ones with the lens that has three vision levels but no line as in bifocals. She was having a hard time making that adjustment, and she took them back after one week of trying to see without feeling dizzy at times. Her optometrist said to her, "In the past, you have been able to look from side to side and up and down by moving your eyes only…glancing, in other words. Now, with these new lenses, you have to be intentional about what you want to see. You can't just move your eyes, you have to move your head and focus on an object."

In the case of needs, you have to look around and focus and then do what you can to help. We were trying to focus everywhere we went and make a list of the needs as we saw them, and, believe me, they were many!

Getting to Know the Albanian People

I was so amazed and touched by the generosity and love shown to us by the Albanian people even though they didn't have much themselves. For instance, one time, when I was visiting our missionary, Theresa Weaver, she suggested I go across the street from her house and visit an old widow who lived there. Of course I did not know the language, but Theresa said it would be OK. I knew enough kind words to say to her, and I would be blessed by my visit, so I went, all by myself. I knew of this widow because our organization had been helping her with food and other needs during the Kosovo crisis, and I really wanted to make her acquaintance personally.

So knowing very little of her language, except maybe "good afternoon, how are you?" I went over to see Gjysha Anna, a sweet widow lady. She brought me inside her little two-room home and sat me down and brought me a cup of thick hot coffee (Turkish coffee) in a tiny little demitasse cup. Thank goodness, it wasn't a mug! She put plenty of sugar in it so I could drink it, and we sipped on the coffee together, and she went to a small cabinet in her living room and pulled out a plate with some little tiny tea cakes that she had made. She made me take one to eat with my coffee, and she mainly sat and smiled and spoke in her language though I knew nothing of what she was saying. I just continuously smiled and said two words I knew that were words of affirmation. They are "po," which means "yes," and "mire" (meer) which means "good."

THE MAKING OF A WONDERFUL LIFE

I was able to tell her I was from Shprese per Boten (Hope for the World) and that I loved her (Te dua shume). And I could tell her Jesus loved her, too, and "God bless you" (Zoti ju bekofte). Whenever she spoke to me, I would try to nod my head from side to side, which in Albania means "yes," not "no," and say "po" (yes). It was so hard to do that! Just try it! Shake your head "no" and say "yes" at the same time. It was nearly impossible! I laughed at myself, and she laughed with me. When I left, she gave me the little cup to take home with me. I did not mean for her to give me anything, but she insisted. She had beautiful flowers blooming in her little courtyard, and I stopped and let her tell me the names of each one. I will never forget my time with Gjysha Anna. There is nothing closer to the heart of God than widows and orphans. I know so because of the many references in scripture and his plan for people to care for them.

When I got back to the missionary's home, I asked her, "Theresa, why would this widow woman go to the trouble to give me coffee and a cake and then give me the cup? Why, she has absolutely nothing of her own!"

Theresa proceeded to tell me that the Albanian people feel that the very worst thing that could happen to them would be for them to have a visitor pass by their way and come to spend time with them, and they do not have anything to give them. They always keep something in their special cupboard just for that visitor. Do you think I was humbled by this experience? You can be very sure I was! To this very day, every time I go to Albania, I come away determined once again to try to practice some of their precious ways in my own home. Lord, please help me!

Another wonderful lesson we have learned from the Albanian people is just how much they value their family and take care of their elderly in the family. In the Albanian culture, whenever the children begin to marry, the first son married will bring his bride to live with his parents. She will then assume much of the workload that her mother-in-law has handled. Then when the next son marries, that first son and wife can move out on their own and the second son and his wife take their place, and so it continues through the family. The last son to marry is to stay with his parents and care for them the rest of their lives. Now, I'm not saying that this is always the case, but it has been a cultural tradition through many years of their history. Most of the houses are built upward with different stories. This enables each of the sons to have their own floor for a home and still live on the property with their parents. This was a custom I found to be very special in Albania. I can't see that working very well in America, can you? Is that a good thing? You decide. That is no doubt why the Albanian people have always preferred to have sons rather than daughters. I always wondered what was their thinking, if no daughters, where would their sons find wives? Things are changing along those lines today in Albania. A lot of our western civilization ways are coming to them. Some good, some not so good.

First Meeting with the Albanian Government

I will never forget Roger telling me about one of the very first meetings he had with the Ministry of Labor and Social Services. It was about the execution of a contract concerning the orphanage in Tirana. He took an interpreter with him, of course, as he could not speak one word in Shqip, and chances were that the Albanian official would not understand one word of English either. I am so glad that was Roger's part of the work and not mine. One very strange thing about their language is that shaking of the head for "yes" and nodding for "no." "Yes" and "no" in the Albanian language are totally opposite from our nodding or shaking of the head. In other words, when they mean "yes," they are in agreement, they are shaking their head back and forth like we would be saying "no" in the English language. And when they mean "no," they give a distinct forward nod, like a real strong show of affirmation in English. But it means "no" in Shqip. Very confusing indeed for us westerners!

That being said, when Roger was in his first meeting that day, and was making known the plans we had to assist the orphans in their country, the Minister of Labor was continually shaking his head back and forth in apparent disagreement.

Roger looked at his interpreter and said, "We may as well leave here. He is disagreeing with everything I'm saying."

The interpreter and the minister both had a great laugh! It was a real ice breaker for them, and they wound up having a very good meeting of the minds and made some wonderful decisions and bonded as friends on that day. As a matter of fact, I must say that although Roger had not had one bit of previous experience meeting with officials of any government before, through the years, they have all truly respected him and become very good friends. It has been a wonderful blessing for me to watch God use him in so many ways in this very different and sometimes difficult arena of our ministry. He is now right at home with the highest dignitaries in Albania. And, really, so am I now that we have been there for so many years.

In fact, I have my own experience involving an Albanian dignitary that I may as well share with you right now before it leaves my mind. We were traveling to Albania one time from America. Our itinerary took us from here to Vienna, Austria, and then on to Albania. It was a time when one of the former prime ministers of Albania, Sali Berisha, was out of office, having been defeated by another party. However, he was still looked at in Albania as a very prominent person. We happened to be in the airport in Vienna, Austria, and at the gate awaiting departure to Albania. Prime Minister Berisha was there as well. I did not realize who he was, but Roger spotted him behind us sitting with his back to us, and he told me who he was. I said to Roger, "Let's go over and meet him," and Roger, of course, refused.

I really wanted to meet Mr. Berisha, but not only that, I wanted to let him know how much we love Albania and love working with the orphans there. I also wanted him to know about Hope for the World and how many years we had been in the country. I loved his hometown of Shkodra and wanted him to know that as well. I went around to him and put out my hand and spoke to him in English (as I knew that he spoke English fluently). I introduced myself to him and told him of our work in Albania. He was very kind and cordial to me, and then I tapped Roger on the back and had him turn around and meet him, too. I know that Roger could have killed me for being so intrusive, but I am a firm believer in the Latin phrase, "carpe diem" (seize the day)!

Sali Berisha was reelected as prime minister in the next election, so I was very glad I could say I had met him personally. I will never forget another prestigious meeting we scheduled with his wife, Dr. Liri Berisha, in Albania when we were really begging the coun-

THE MAKING OF A WONDERFUL LIFE

try to give us some property where we could begin a center for the teenaged orphans who were made to leave the orphanage after the eighth grade. It seemed that these kids had been so overlooked and were given such a really bad shake in life, and our hearts were burdened for them. Dr. Berisha had founded what was known as "The Albanian Children Foundation." It was dedicated to helping abandoned, orphaned, poor, and destitute children. We knew that as a medical doctor, she focused on a desire to treat and cure children suffering from different congenital disorders or other severe pathologies such as autism and psychoneurological problems. We really believed that if we could get some quality time with her, she might be able to persuade her husband and other powers that be, to let us have that particular piece of property to help these teenaged orphans. This meeting was in September of 2008.

We knew that many of the orphans, if given half a chance, would go on and finish high school and maybe even go into the university, if they just had a place where people loved them, encouraged them, assisted them in their studies, and mentored them. The university was free to any student who could qualify academically. The purpose of our visit to Mrs. Berisha was to ask her about a certain piece of property we knew the government owned and was not using. It had been vacant for years and was in a very nice location along the ocean side. It could easily have served as a special home for the teens.

I never will forget that meeting. We had made sure our president and founder of Hope for the World in America, Mr. Jimmy Franks, and his wife, Janice, came to sit in on this meeting. Of course, we also had our in-country president, Perparim Demcellari, and a staff director, Fredi Zefi, in attendance with us that day. Rodney and Kimberly Tucker, a very special couple from Greensboro, North Carolina, were with us on our trip that time, so we were happy to include them in this meeting as well. We had quite an entourage with us as we visited Mrs. Berisha that day.

On a personal note, I remember I was a little perplexed at just what to wear to such a meeting. This would be my first "sit-down meeting" with any of the high officials in Albania. I had only brought one skirt with me for Sunday services, so that was my only choice of apparel for the day. It wasn't actually a "dress for success" look, but it was the only dress I had with me, so that was what I wore. Of all things, when we came to the meeting and were seated, I was right beside Dr. Berisha. Yes, I was just a little bit nervous, but I tried to act like I truly had it all together, and actually I enjoyed our time with her. She listened about the plight of the orphan children. She appreciated the many years we had been there, since 1992, working to help the orphans in Albania, but there was no indication from her that her government would be doing anything at all to help us assist these teenaged orphans. Now, she didn't say they wouldn't help either, so we just came away from that meeting hoping and at least knowing that someone at her level knew our hearts and our desire for them to help us with that piece of property, and that was the end of the matter. Hope for the World also made a nice donation to her cause of working with autistic children in Albania, as we knew of many children with autism who lived in the orphanages.

Someone from Dr. Berisha's office told us about a man in New York City who had been known to give generous donations to things pertaining to the needs of the children in Albania and that he had been a part of helping her cause. They suggested that we make an appointment and go to see him at some point in time to see if he would help us financially for this project for the teens.

Well, we were not to be discouraged, so Jimmy and Janice Franks and Roger and I made plans to take a trip to New York that coming December and see this gentleman to whom we had been referred. Our trip was twofold actually. We decided we would love to go and see some of the Christmas shows while we were there as none of us had ever been.

When we got back to the States, Roger allowed a little time to pass, and then he made a phone call to this gentleman, who was definitely Italian, by his name. Roger spoke with someone in his office, telling them about our work in Albania and asking for a meeting. We told them we had plans to come to New York in December, so a date was set for us to have lunch with this man.

The December date arrived. We flew to New York City and were staying around 42nd Street and Broadway. An interesting side note, I just remembered that the valet who helped us to our room at the hotel was an Albanian young man! He was so surprised when we asked him his country of origin and that we had all been to his country and knew so much about it. We were able to witness to him and make a good friend of him throughout our stay there. We were shown by a map that the place we were to meet the benevolent man was not too many blocks from where we were staying, so we decided to walk. It turned out to be further than we had thought, and it was colder than cold in New York in December. We went to the office of the gentleman and met with his personal assistant who then took us on another hike to the place we were to meet for lunch.

When we arrived at the place for the lunch meeting, we took a stairway to the entrance which was below street level. We were actually let into a private club. It made us feel like we were entering something that might be a part of the Italian Mafia. Who knows? We had never been taken to such a place for a meal before. We were met by the gentleman we had come to see, and he immediately looked at Roger and noted that he was wearing a turtleneck sweater with his blazer, but no dress shirt and tie. Now, Brother Jimmy was dressed "right" with a suit and tie. He then asked one of the assistants to get a tie for Roger. He was wearing a gray turtleneck and a navy blazer. They gave him a burgundy tie, and he had to put it around his turtleneck sweater and wear it during the meal. Well, we were all so tickled and wanted to laugh out loud but were actually afraid to do so. We didn't know where we were or who we were with, and it was all very strange indeed.

We were taken from the dark entrance hall into a very dimly lit dining room with no windows, as we were underground. We were all seated at a round table for eight. There were no more tables, no more people. Were we eating with the Godfather? The gentleman's wife was present, another lady who was his secretary, and the gentleman who was his personal assistant. The older gentleman we had come to see sat between Roger and Brother Jimmy. Janice and I sat where we could more easily speak with the women. Speak about what, we had no clue. We had no idea really how we were going to relate. Talk about fish out of water? That was us. What made it harder for us too is that on the inside we were quivering, both from a little fright, and then also from trying to stifle our chuckles at Roger with his "formal" turtleneck.

Thank God for Brother Jimmy, he was never at a loss for words. He sort of broke the ice for us by beginning to tell his story of his first time to ever visit Albania. Part of it was humorous, and they laughed with us, so that put a little relaxation into the air. Then after Jimmy talked a while, we could see that this gentleman was truly being touched by his story, and at times he was wiping his eyes as they teared up. Then we began to pray within ourselves that God would touch their hearts and bring these people to salvation. We really didn't know what to expect, to tell you the truth.

Roger was the one to bring our need of a place for the teen-aged orphans into the conversation. The man seemed very interested and, like I said, even had some of his own life experiences to tell us that seemed to equate with some of the stories from the lives of our orphan children. He had come from very poor beginnings in Sicily. And here he was now, a very big-time operator in New York. Now how he had made his money, we have no idea! The meal was very lengthy as there were many different courses and no hurry to clear one off and bring the next. Oh, it was *fine dining* at its best. They certainly did not spare anything and actually rolled out the red carpet for us on that day. As a matter of fact, the carpet may have actually been red in the entrance hall. I'm just not really sure about that as I try to recall.

By the time we came out from our lunch, it was nearly dark in New York City. We got a cab back to our hotel, and though we had made a great plea for help for the orphans, we never heard one word from these people. So now, you might say, there were two strikes as far as making pitches on behalf of the orphans, to both the Albanian government and the Italian "elite." What it truly showed us once more is that God's work is, and has always been, provided for by God's people. It always had happened that way in the past, and it looked very much like that was the way God would have it to be in the present and future as well.

We did not lose hope, and we did not give up, but we did pray even harder and more fervently that somehow, and in some way, God would allow us to buy property in Albania to be able to start a Hope Center to give hope for the future to the orphans of Albania.

A Hole in Her Heart

One of the early blessings that we can never forget was on an early visit Roger made to the preschool orphanage in Shkoder not long after we had begun working there. He was just getting to know the director, Maria, and other workers who had told him about one of the little girls, Fitneta, who had been born with a hole in her heart. At that time, the medical facilities in Albania were not equipped sufficiently to handle a lot of procedures such as heart surgeries. They could diagnose the problems, and there were very smart physicians in the country, but it was a matter of not having the equipment needed. Roger was very burdened about this little girl and told them he was going to come back home and see if there was anything we could do from America to try to help her.

He was on the plane leaving Albania that time when he noticed a group of what appeared to be medical professionals boarding the plane with a group of children of various ages. There were also some other adults, maybe parents or caregivers in the group. That plane was going from Albania to Austria which was Roger's connecting airport.

After they were in the air, Roger struck up a conversation with one of the men who happened to be a medical doctor from a hospital in Austria. When Roger inquired about the children they had in their company, he was told that these were children from Albanian families who had some serious physical problems that required surgeries that could not be performed in Albania at that time.

Roger then asked the good doctor if they had ever done any of these operations on any orphan children from Albania, to which he replied, "No, we had not." Roger then asked if they would be open to helping a little orphan girl who had a hole in her heart. He told Roger that they certainly would be open to doing so, and he gave Roger his contact information so that we could communicate with the proper office in Austria to see what could be worked out.

When Roger got home that time, he was so excited and called it a direct answer to his prayers as he had been praying that the Lord would provide a way to help this little girl. We got busy right away by email with our people in Albania, getting all the necessary medical information to the hospital in Austria and planning for a time that this might be accomplished. They told us they would also need someone from Albania who could speak English to accompany Fitneta and plan to stay there with her during her recovery period and then bring her back to Albania.

It did not take many weeks for all of this to be arranged, and next thing we knew, little Fitneta was taken to Austria, had the surgery to mend the hole in her heart, and brought back to the orphanage. Everyone was so thrilled to know that she could now live a normal healthy life. This girl lived in the orphanages all through her grade school years, and when it was time for her to start into high school, we had our Tag Center for Teens opened (which you will read about later in this book). Fitneta became one of our first residents there. She had accepted Christ as her Savior as a little girl, and she grew spiritually all the years she spent in the Tag Center. She was such a blessing to all of us, and every year when she would celebrate another birthday, we would all rejoice that God had miraculously provided medical help for her as that little girl years before when she had the hole in her heart.

The greatest blessing of all, however, was that Fitneta had found Christ as her personal Savior, and he had filled the spiritual hole in her heart.

First Granddaughter

As we were just getting greatly involved in our work in Albania, and as Buddy and the boys were really doing well in their Christian music careers, we found out that Kerri and Buddy were expecting their very first baby, and guess what, they were expecting our very *first granddaughter*! You may sometimes think that after you already have two grandchildren and they have been a big part of your lives for about seven years, it would be *no big deal* to hear that you are going to be grandparents all over again! But not so! For one thing, we had seen our daughter become a mommy and saw what a great little mommy she was! But we had absolutely no idea how it would be to see our son become a daddy! And to beat that, the daddy of a little *girl*? Oh my goodness! How special was this going to be?

Well, this news was so exciting to everyone in our family! We had been *all about boys* since the births of Brady in 1989 and then Austin in 1993. Now here it was in 1995, and we were expecting our very first granddaughter. Now, it's not that we didn't already love Kerri to death and think that she was the most beautiful daughter-in-law inside and out, but just knowing that she was carrying our very first precious little princess truly endeared her to us as never before. You see, Buddy and Kerri had been married for five years already, and though we never said it, we were truly wondering when and "if" we were going to have any grandchildren from this couple. But we know it was all in God's timing, and we can look back now and see how good it was for them to wait those five years.

The time seemed to go by pretty fast, for us. Maybe not so fast for Kerri. However, she certainly did pick the perfect season for her pregnancy to mature. She went through her last trimester in the winter months of October, November, and December. We really thought we'd have a little Christmas "Carol," and then we thought we would have the first baby of the New Year of 1996, but God allowed Victoria Scarlett Mullins to come into the world around 10:30 a.m. on January 2, 1996, at the Williamson Medical Center in Franklin, Tennessee, weighing seven pounds and eleven ounces, so we would all be through celebrating both Christmas and the New Year and could give all of our energy and attention to celebrating the birth of this beautiful granddaughter. What a wonderful day that was for all of the Mullins family as well as the King family! I think I have told you that Kerri was an "only child," so this was such a momentous occasion for her parents, Tommy and Merleene King. They lived in Gadsden, Alabama. We lived in Stockbridge, Georgia, at that time, so that meant both sets of grandparents lived *too far away*.

When I think back on this now, I can really appreciate Kerri and Buddy even more as new parents with no grandparents near them, raising their first little girl all "on their own," so to speak. If it had not been for April Willett, I really don't know how Kerri would have made it. April was just enough younger than Kerri and without any children yet that she could be there with Kerri and for her and Victoria while her husband, Wes, and Buddy were both out on the road in their group known as "Sunday Drive" at that time. What a tremendous help April was! She always kept a set of Kerri's keys to her house, and I know what a tremendous help she was to Kerri in every way imaginable! Taking care of Tori, helping around the house, you name it! April was there and really was the greatest friend to Kerri. She and Wes still are their *very best friends*. God is so good to provide for the needs we have as we go through life. Friends stepping in when there are no grandparents around, how special was that? It makes me love April more all over again. She came from our church, Glen Haven, and we had known her and her grandparents, as well as her parents, for years before she and Wes ever met. She comes from a great family who love the Lord with their whole heart.

Well, Victoria Scarlett was quite the little girl! We all so enjoyed her and loved getting to see her in all of the beautiful phases of little girlhood! Her Neena, that's Kerri's mom's name given to her by her grandchildren, being the talented seamstress she was, began very early making the most beautiful frilly little dresses and hats for Tori. Tori has the *biggest* dark brown eyes and dark brown hair. Tori has used her considerable singing and acting talents constantly to entertain us as well as many, many others. She really came into the world as a little professional entertainer I believe!

We would always love it when we could go to Nashville and see Tori in one of her church musicals or plays in which she was performing or just simply standing in a row with other kids and singing her heart out! She'd always be modeling a beautiful costume creation by Neena and usually with a hat to match. With Buddy operating their video camera, if we hadn't seen her good enough from our seat in the church, we could all get the real "close-up" shots he had taken of her when we viewed the video at home.

Victoria always was our little entertainer. From the time she was big enough to talk, she began singing! Of course, it was almost a given being that her mom and dad, grandparents, Aunt Cindy, friends, and neighbors were all singers. It is just in her genes.

When Tori came along, Austin was already two years of age, and Brady was six. By the time she was three, this trio could put on some pretty awesome after-supper shows whenever they got together. As a matter of fact, I believe Tori was doing her own solo gigs at home and at Papa and Neena's house as well as our house whenever she came to spend the night. I had a closet full of high heels, big colorful scarves and swimsuit wraps, and hats ranging from huge hats with wide brims to the cute little golf caps in various colors. These worked great for her showstoppers, and she could put together quite the costumes.

It's quite ironic that I was writing about Victoria at *this particular* time and on *this particular* day. She is now nineteen years old, and we just returned from their home in Santa Rosa Beach, Florida, where she had a starring role in the theatrical production of "Oklahoma" at the Mattie Kelly Arts Center at Northwest Florida

State College in Niceville. And she is standing in line right at this very moment in Savannah, Georgia, at the *American Idol* auditions. Who knows what will come of that? I have just been notified that she has already passed round one and round two and has one more round to go in front of the cameras and the production staff. If she makes it there, then her next round will be in front of the stars. Go, Tori! So you see what I meant when I said she came out of the womb as a born entertainer?

All the way through her high school years in Florida, she was cast in every high school drama, and in her senior year, she had the leading role as Fanny Bryce in the musical comedy, *Funny Girl*. She has kept us entertained all her life so far. Her talents really glow as she sings worship and praise tunes with her family. She and her cousin, Austin, make a great duo, too, as do she and her sister, Olivia.

Right now, I am writing during the month of January 2016, and the final season of *American Idol* has just started. I wasn't able to tell this for a number of months, as I had actually had to sign a contract that kept me from telling anything at all about what I knew to be happening for Victoria with American Idol, but now I am able to tell it. She actually won the auditions in Savannah, Georgia, this past summer where there were over three thousand who entered that competition. She made it through three different auditions on that day which meant she would have one more audition in Atlanta, Georgia, in September. She was allowed to bring six family members and friends with her. She brought her mom; her sister, Olivia; her cousin, Austin; her friend, Suzanne; and both of us grandmothers. I remember it was on a Sunday. We got up very early as we had to be there by about 7:00 a.m. in downtown Atlanta at a hotel.

We were all so excited! It was still dark when we arrived and sort of cool that morning as we had to line up out on the street awaiting all the instructions. When we finally went inside to the holding room, I think there were probably about fifty to sixty different ones there who had won their previous auditions and were ready to go before the judges who were Harry Connick Jr., J.Lo, and Keith Urban. We waited and waited in great anticipation. Different ones would break out into playing and singing in the holding room. Tori and Austin and Livi even got involved as Austin brought his guitar in with him and Livi had a ukulele. It was fun actually, and the time went pretty fast although we were there all day long before Tori actually went in for her audition.

There were cameras everywhere! They videoed every single thing that went on in that place that day! You know, they have a great show to produce, so they don't want anything to be overlooked or missed that might be something they'd like to include. We were so excited when Tori went in to do her audition! We all waited outside that door where she would come through either delighted or dejected. Well, she came bursting through the door waving her gold ticket to Hollywood! She jumped into Austin's arms! He swung her around, and then we all took our turns hugging her and congratulating her! This was truly a *big* moment for all of us, but especially for Tori.

It wasn't easy not being able to tell people or put it out on Facebook or any social media. We had to keep it tightly locked within the family. I think it was one of the hardest things we'd ever had to do, especially us grandmothers! You know how we like to brag on our grandkids!

In the final season of *American Idol*, we did see her face a couple of times. Though we didn't get to see her audition, they did televise her bursting through the door, waving her golden ticket, and all of us were on TV as we high-fived her and Austin caught her as she jumped in his arms. Then there was also a little minute they showed of her talking to the crew briefly about her plans to do her best before the judges that day. She didn't stay long in the competition once she got to Hollywood, but a couple of her girlfriends from home had taken a week's vacation in Hollywood and had a hotel room where she spent the entire week and had a great time.

She was not really too disappointed as her goal was to get to go to Hollywood. She went right on with her life as normal when she got back home. In fact, it freed her up to continue her plans to make an extended visit to Albania in the fall of 2016 to see if God has some special plans for her in the world of foreign missions. Her talent will be used of God and for God as long as she will give it all to him. That is always our prayer concerning our grandchildren. By the way, Tori returned from spending a full month in Albania on a mission for the orphans. She spent the first 2 1/2 weeks in Shkoder, living with the Zefi family who have worked with HFTW for fifteen years. She helped mainly in the baby orphanage but was also a part of life in all of the orphanages. Her final days were spent at our Hope Center for Teens and being toured around a lot of Albania by our very efficient secretary/tour guide, Ledina Rabdishta. They actually bonded like sisters. She had a wonderful time and got back here just in time for Thanksgiving.

Backtracking a little, I briefly mentioned above that during the time that Tori was a baby, Buddy and Wes were still singing and traveling together. They still had the same group intact as when Roger was traveling and singing with them. It was Mark and Wes Willett, Paul Lancaster, Joel Huggins on lead guitar, Marvin Sims on the drums, and Buddy. They were then known as "Sunday Drive," and their music style was very contemporary. They were getting some great tours with Evangelist Josh McDowell in some amazing events for the youth of America. They also were fronting in the "Stained Glass Tour" of Clay Crosse and Jaci Velasquez as well as Mark Lowry's "Mouth in Motion Tour." They made two recordings as "Sunday Drive." One was named after their group, simply, "Sunday Drive," and the other one was "Doors Open Wide." They were kept pretty busy in this group and worked very hard.

On many days that Buddy was not traveling, he tried to help Kerri by taking care of Victoria while she was working for their cousin, DeAnne Cotthoff, in the real estate business. The great thing about Kerri working for DeAnne was that her office was in her home, so Kerri could bring Victoria to work with her, and she more or less raised her there at De's home office from the time she was a little baby. Buddy said that he toted Tori around so much with him in Nashville that even if he wasn't known by name by many, he became known in the music world as "that singer with the baby." They would often see Buddy appear for lunches and various music industry gatherings carrying Tori in her little car seat. She and her daddy really bonded early in her life.

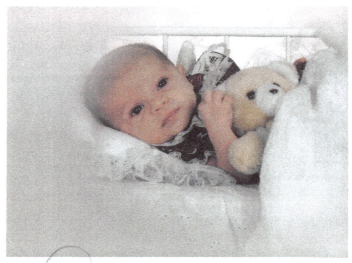

Victoria Scarlet Mullins born January 2, 1996
A joy and an entertainer from the very beginning.

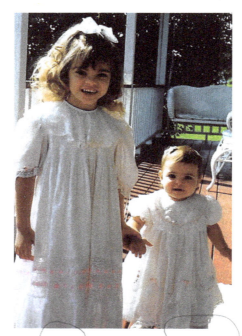

Big Sister Victoria with little Sister Olivia
Wearing some of those dresses made by their "Neena".

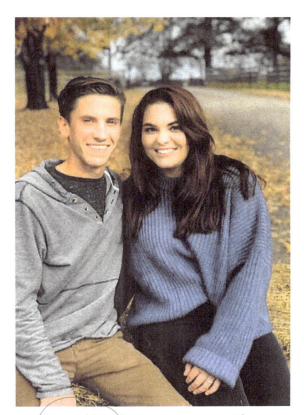

Tori and Matthew—Engagement Photo

A Great Missionary and Friend, David Hosaflook

Interviewed by Cherie

Since we have been working in Albania, we have come to know and appreciate very much a young man named David Hosaflook. He has actually been a missionary to Albania a little longer than we have. His ministry has been first and foremost in Shkodra, Albania, where he began the Bible Baptist Church. He has been very instrumental in the discipleship of our Albanian staff as their pastor and mentor for many years. He and his wife, Kristi, have been, and continue to be, a great blessing to Albanians. I had asked him if he would mind sharing a little about his early days in Albania as a young single man and then bring us up to date with what God is doing through him at the present time in Albania. He suggested that I pose some specific questions to him and let him answer them. I would like at this time to share with you this interview with David.

David, tell me about your calling to the mission field.

I felt at eight years old that God was leading me into missions. My calling was reconfirmed during mission trips to Mexico at age fifteen or sixteen. After graduating from Bible college, I went to Mexico again and was also invited to go to Albania in 1992 with Pastor David Janney, of Orlando Baptist Church, who was one of the founders of HFTW. I accepted the invitation and went to Albania. I lived at the orphanage that summer and worked with the children and helped them to learn about Jesus. I went thinking it would just be for the summer, not realizing it would be for many years. I am still in Albania today.

What did you do with Hope for the World?

In 1992, HFTW was just getting started on the ground in Albania. There was a big learning curve for all involved with HFTW. The country was in a mess, there was a crisis for food, and the orphanage in Tirana appeared in shambles, literally in squalid conditions and very unsanitary. It was probably worse than the condition of the country itself which was very bad at that time.

We mostly spent time with the children, making relationships. We organized some youth camps for children at the beach at Golem, sort of a holiday place for the kids although it was in very bad condition, too. We told the children the gospel, and many of them accepted Christ. I still have many signatures in my Bible of the children who were saved that summer at the camp in Golem.

Tell me how you met Kristi and about how she adapted to life in Albania.

I met Kristi in 1995 at a missions conference at Orlando Baptist. She came and visited Albania in 1996, and we were married in 1997. I actually had left Albania in January of 1997, and immediately after that, Albania blew up in anarchy due to the pyramid crisis. So, yes, I was already a missionary in Albania when I met Kristi. She was very interested in the work of HFTW because of her connection to Orlando Baptist Church. I don't know exactly when the leadership of HFTW in Albania passed to Roger and Cherie Mullins, but that was a welcome transfer for me because Roger had a gift for administration and organization. He also had a passion and commitment focused exclusively on HFTW Albania and raising the necessary funds to meet the budget and to make sure that all of the funds were properly used and the programs were well maintained. It seemed that although HFTW had a very difficult beginning in Albania's development as a country, it was finally getting the attention that was needed. I really appreciated Roger and his work.

As far as how my wife, Kristi, adjusted to life in Albania, it was very hard. When we returned in 1997, Albania was still in a state of unrest and war with bullets and bombs going off, so she had some real hardships as a young lady with several life-changing events going on at the same time. Her stress levels would be clinically off the charts due to the move, a cross-cultural move, a cross-lingual move, where she didn't understand the language. Of course, just being married is always a life-changing event. She was then being thrown into an environment that was very traumatic with the unrest that was going on in Albania. It was very difficult for her, but God gave her rest and strength, and she is a hero to me to have done all that.

Hosaflook family adoptions

(Editor's note: The Hosaflooks have three children born to them, besides these that David speaks of that they have adopted while living in Albania.)

We are pleased that the Lord has allowed us to adopt two children as well as take in a young lady who had grown up in the orphanage but then did not have anywhere to go after she left. All three of those children have been a great blessing to our family, and our biological children have been a blessing to their adopted siblings. There were two legal adoptions we were able to, by God's grace, get through the Albanian courts. One was an almost two-year-old little girl who was from the Shkodra baby orphanage, and she is now grown up, and what a blessing she has been to our family. We have recently adopted another young lady who was nearly sixteen years old. She spent most of her life in the orphanage and didn't have anywhere to go. As we began advocating for her to try to find some parents, we realized that her time was so limited, that even if we found someone, there wouldn't be enough time for the adoption to go through, and she would soon be in the orphan dormitories. That is a synonym for saying "being on the street" and vulnerable to the worst vermin of society. So we realized that we had enough time to adopt her if we just worked quickly. The Lord led us to do that, and we are very pleased to have adopted her as well. We find ourselves blessed as we have tried to bless them.

When did you begin the Bible Baptist Church in Shkodra?

Toward the end of 1993 and into 1994, the church spent a lot of time meeting in the preschool orphanage in Shkodra. This was just like the Tirana Bible Baptist Church which began its meetings in the Tirana orphanage where I was very involved along with Jeff Bartel, who would end up staying in that church as pastor when I moved to Shkodra. In 1994, I was a missionary pastor, and as soon as I could, I began transferring leadership to the Albanian believers who were coming to faith in Christ. We are very thankful for them and how God has equipped them to do a work that is indigenous today, and they continue to serve faithfully and fruitfully.

Personal note from Cherie: This church is the one that has been so very effective and instrumental in the spiritual growth of our staff workers in Shkodra. Also, they have reached out to the orphans and to the workers in the government orphanages in Shkodra. It plays a great role in Christian leadership for all who have been a part of Hope for the World, and we thank God for this great church. Some of our staff hold strong leadership positions in this church at this time. Many have been saved here, and it is truly a lighthouse in Albania in that area.

What did Albania look like when you first came?

It looked very much like a typical communist country with all of the sort of square blocks of apartments that all look the same. If you look at North Korea today, there is a lot of similarity. There are very few, if any, buildings taller than six stories. The rural areas of the country were very depressed and very poor. There were no big tractors and other agricultural equipment. There was not much more than a hoe and a scythe. It was just a very poor country. Now, of course, with the fall of communism, that has all changed. Roads have been built and better bridges, and the infrastructure is as though we have actually just skipped a generation.

Could you tell me a memorable story concerning someone's conversion in Albania?

That is hard because everyone's conversion story is memorable from the orphans who heard the gospel in Tirana sitting with us on the steps of the orphanage, or watching a sunset by the seaside in Golem at the camp. Each young person that expressed his faith in Christ is memorable to me. In Shkodra, the first one to accept Christ was Arben, who is now the pastor of the church there. I just remember walking and talking and walking and talking for hours with him as he really wanted to understand what the Gospel was, especially as it contrasted with his religious background, so the first ones are always memorable. Shortly after Arben's conversion, Beni brought Fredi Zefi over to my house, and he told me that he had been sharing with Fredi what I had been telling him and Fredi would like to know more. Fredi was probably already a believer when he was brought to my house, but I remember him praying and it being sort of confirmed right there in my apartment. And then Fredi's brother, Astrit, and the list goes on and on of so many who have been rescued from darkness and saved by the grace of the Lord Jesus Christ.

How did you get to be so fluent in the Albanian language?

The Albanian language is an ancient language, and it is not related to any other language. It is a branch all of its own in the Indo-European languages. I became fluent in Albanian by immersing myself into the Albanian culture. I didn't have a lot of people to talk to in English, and I worked hard with dictionaries. There was not a good course of Albanian study for foreigners, so I really learned a lot from the orphans and then found private tutors that I could go to and ask for help with things I was struggling with as I began to look at some Albanian books.

I remember just reading Bible verses over and over out loud again and again so that I could see, pronounce, and hear the Albanian language all at the same time, and of course, doing so with Bible verses was very helpful as I began to use Bible verses on a daily basis in my discussions with people. So, over the years, I got more tutors who were at higher levels, but really the key was immersion into the language.

Please tell me about the book you have written.

It is actually a book which a man named Marlin Barletti wrote in 1504. Barletti was an Albanian. He is considered to be the first Albanian to ever have written a book that we know about. His book was about the siege of Shkodra and Mehmed the Conqueror, who had defeated Constantinople (Istanbul) in 1453. It's the story of his coming to Albania in 1478 to take Shkodra. Now, this man had been opposed for many years by Albania's national hero, Skanderbeg, but Skanderbeg died in 1468, and that brought great joy to the Ottoman Empire because they thought they could just run over to Albania without being contested. Of course, Albania wasn't their goal. Their goal was to take Western Europe and actually defeat Rome like they had defeated Constantinople.

They weren't expecting that there would be a remarkable resistance in one of the key remaining cities to be conquered, Shkodra. The Shkodrans were there, Albanians and some other nationalities, and some Venetians as well. The Venetians were the Ottoman's enemies and were Catholics. So the Catholic Venetians and the Catholic Albanians fought very intensely against the Ottomans as the Ottomans besieged the Castle of Shkodra. It was quite a bloody battle, and in the end, the Albanians held out against the Ottomans, and Mehmed the Conqueror never stepped foot inside the city. But later in a peace deal with Venice, Shkodra was sort of given over to the Ottomans, and that brought great joy to the Ottomans, and immediately after that, they began attacking Italy, the Italian peninsula of Otranto.

This is a remarkable event in history that very few historians know much about. In fact, it was so rarely known that when I reached out to top professors of history such as Cambridge history professor David Abulafia, FBA, he recognized the significance of the event and was so welcoming of the new English translation of this book that he wrote a historical introduction to it. That was quite an honor, so with this kind of gravitas that this book has, I have been given opportunities to lecture on the events of the Christian Albanian resistance to the Ottoman Empire and about Marlin Barletti's contribution to literature and to history.

It is especially interesting that in some of the Albanian territories outside of Albania, such as Macedonia and Kosovo, where the overwhelming majority of the people are Muslim today, some of them look back at their roots and say, "Wait a minute, we were Christians before we were Muslims," so maybe it's not such an un-Albanian thing to think about Jesus Christ and consider his claims and consider the Gospel. I let them make that conclusion on their own. But during the course of some of these lectures, some of these Albanian professors said, "You know, David, we don't know so much about Protestant evangelical history and the contributions that the British Bible Society and the American Mission Board, started by Adoniram Judson and his group, made. How did they help Albania? How did they help us with our language and our education?" It's really an amazing thing to realize that the British Bible Society developed the Albanian language to a large degree. Not exclusively, but certainly they were the ones publishing the books. There were hundreds of years of Christianity among the Albanian people, but not until the first quarter of the nineteenth century did the Albanians get published copies of the Word of God in their own language, and that was due to the work of evangelical Christians. Some Albanians go so far as to say that without that work, there might not be an Albania today because, remember, just a little over one hundred years ago, there was no Albania. It was part of the Ottoman Empire, and as the Ottoman Empire began to crumble in the late 1800s and early 1900s, other Balkan nations around today's Albania were becoming very bold and wanting to take the Albanian lands for their own. Albania did not have one common religion to bind them together, so really the only thing that bound them together was their language. But if their language was not developed, written, studied, and embraced by the Albanian people, it really could not be viable as a nation at all. So, really, with the contributions of the missionary community, even though their intentions were predominantly to share the Gospel of Jesus Christ and enable Albanians to read the Bible, as a secondary benefit, the Albanian language was developed. This has given me an interesting platform to develop this history more and many others have been studying this, and so a few years ago, I began talking to other historians of the movement, and we developed an institute for these kinds of studies. The website for that is www.instituti.org, and with that, we are just putting out on an academic level a lot of the writing of the movers and shakers of the evangelical Protestant movement. In the past four years, we have published seventeen books on Albanian Christian history.

(I truly appreciate David for taking the time to write this interesting history for me in my book. All of these people who I am including in my book have had a big part in laying the groundwork for us upon which our ministry in Albania has been built.)

I hope that you are finding very helpful and interesting what has been written here by others.

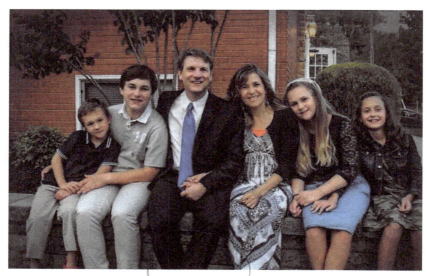

David Hosaflook Family

First Assignment with Hope For the World

Approval of Theresa Weaver as a Missionary

Since Roger had been officially appointed by the governing board of Hope for the World as the director of operations in Albania, there were many new duties that fell under this title. One of them was that we were to interview any would-be missionary applicants who thought they wanted to go as full-time missionaries to Albania. Now, don't get me wrong, but people were not standing in line or knocking on our door daily telling us they wanted to go. But whoever made contact with us and stated that they'd like to go to Albania had to make an appointment to meet with us and let us have an extensive interview with them so we could share with them a lot of information about Albania that they could not get off of the internet from Wikipedia.

I never will forget the very first missionary applicant who contacted us. Her name was Theresa Weaver from Orlando, Florida. We were going to that area anyway, on other business, so we arranged to meet with her at a restaurant for lunch. I believe it was at Ruby Tuesday's. I'll never forget her. She was a short and very petite little lady with a huge, huge smile! She was full of life and had a very bubbly personality. She had been teaching school in the public school system to special ed students. That in itself spoke volumes to me. We did not have a long list of cut and dried questions to go through with her. We mainly needed to have her give us her personal testimony of her salvation and then her experience of service in the Lord's work. We wanted to know about his calling on her life and her plans for her support if she were to go to Albania. We suggested to her that she first plan to go to Albania for at least one month to see if she could adjust to the culture and to solidify her calling to that country and those people. She had a lot of experience with children from her teaching career, so it would be a given that she could fit nicely with children in the orphanages. She planned to learn the language right there on the field as there was really no other place here in America for her to learn to speak Shqip. I don't even recall if there were any courses available for purchase to learn the language at home. Now, of course, there are several on the market. Rather than talk any further about Theresa, I will let her share her testimony in her own words in answer to questions I asked her.

Theresa Weaver

Interviewed by Cherie Mullins

When did you first go into Albania?

I first came into Albania in 1993 for the longest, "short-term missions" trip ever in my life, three months! I came with my church, Orlando Baptist.

And how were you called to serve in Albania?

Ever since I was saved, I had felt the tugging of the Holy Spirit in my heart to be a foreign missionary. In 1994, the Lord directed me to go to H.E.A.R.T, a missionary training camp in Lake Wales, Florida, to learn how to live in a third-world country. All of us students were seeking the Lord as to where he wanted us to go. I had put out several "fleeces" to the Lord as I wrote to different missionaries, but all the positions were closed. Our church was heavily involved with Albania at the time, and that year, during our annual missions' conference, my pastor asked me if I would pray about going to Albania and working in the orphanage in Shkoder. I told him I didn't have to pray anymore because that was the answer to my prayers! I had been heavily praying about our church's work in Albania because I was the church's missionary liaison and also was sponsoring an orphan there.

What was your area of work with Hope for the World?

My first job with HFTW was to share Christ's love with the preschool orphans, the staff, and the director as well as keep our valuable sponsors connected with the orphans and vice versa. I was to learn the language and the culture (and simply try to survive!). I actually started working full-time in the preschool orphanage in Shkoder in the summer of 1995. I also helped the director with any projects to enhance the living conditions in the orphanages and in the lives of those precious children. I taught God's valuable word and even Christian songs to the children. This was the very first time in the staff's and children's lives to hear the gospel or even to sing songs of praise to their Creator and Savior. What a wonderful privilege. Along with the work at the orphanage, I assisted Pastor David Hosaflook in reaching the ladies for Christ in the church work. He was single at the time and needed a female to help him with part of the ministry.

How did you learn the language?

The Lord gave me the Albanian language. I am writing a book entitled *New Tongues*, and the following is an excerpt from my book:

In November 1995 (I wrote next to Mark 16:17 in my Bible), "And these signs shall follow them that believe; In my name shall they cast out devils; they shall speak with new tongues." The new tongue I had was Shqip. I prayed that the Lord would help me learn this language. In the early 1990s in Albania, it was hard to find someone who knew English, so I didn't have a language teacher. I carried around a backpack which always had my English/Albanian and Albanian/English dictionaries in it. I remember going to the little "hole in the wall" store wanting deodorant and having to pull out my dictionaries and point to the word deodorant. In Shkoder, they called it "under the arm," but in the Albanian dictionary, it said "deodorant." After much work and sign language, the storekeeper brought me the deodorant. Life went on like that with my dictionaries. I lived with an Albanian widow named Nene Maria, and she helped me a bit with my language. She'd go to the door, open it, and say, "Hape daren." She'd close it and say, "Mbylle daren." I'd go open the door and try to repeat what she'd said. The Holy Spirit was helping me remember because I was thirty-three years old, and this was the hardest language I've ever learned! I knew Spanish, French, and sign language, but this one really was getting the better of me. I needed the Lord's help more than ever in my life as far as learning a language was concerned.

Around 4:00 p.m. each day, I'd hurry home for my "language lesson." We'd get electricity, and I'd turn the TV on to watch a channel that had old John Wayne movies dubbed in Italian with Albanian subtitles. I remember watching John Wayne movies growing up so knew what was happening. The subtitles helped me read in Shqip, and I'd look up a word I saw repeatedly to find out what it meant. I'd also study with my *Colloquial Albanian* language book which came with a cassette. I studied three hours a day. For the first five months, I was speaking enough to make myself understood in daily living, but when it came to sharing the Gospel and talking about deep spiritual needs, it was becoming too frustrating for me to bear. I tried not speaking English with the Albanians who knew some and wanted me to teach them because I needed to learn their language. I finally reached my limit one day when there were some Albanians in my house visiting Nene Maria, and I couldn't concentrate on what they were talking about any more. Frustration drove me to gather the coffee cups and go into the kitchen, which was in the same room as the guests, and wash them. As I washed, streams of tears rolled down my face as I poured out my heart to the Lord telling him how much I needed to have the Albanian language so I could share his priceless Gospel with the lost. I was ready to give up and go to the States to share the glorious truth with my fellow countrymen if he didn't give me the Albanian language.

I had read many stories of missionaries smuggling Bibles into different communist countries, and at the borders God miraculously gave them the same border language which was unknown to the missionary, but he/she spoke it and was sent on their merry way. I begged the Lord to give me the language if he thought I was worthy of it so that I could honor him and share him with others. At that moment, my ears, which had seemed to have ear plugs in them, were unplugged! The guests in the room continued to talk, and I could tell when one word finished and the other word began. The Holy Spirit opened the door of my understanding and gave meaning to those sentences. He also loosened my tongue so that I'd be able to somewhat pronounce the very long words they have. I was caught up in the moment of this miracle and started jumping up and down with joy that he gave me their language! These people are a reserved people group, and I was jumping up and down saying, "I understand you! I understand you!" I have no idea what they did or said after that because I was caught up in the spirit of my own delight. The Lord of languages gave me this gift. Unfortunately, I only asked him for the language so that I could share the Gospel with this people. I had to continue working for the rest of the language, and in 1997 and 1998, I did pay people to be my teachers. I wish I would have asked the Lord for *all* the Albanian language so that I wouldn't have to work hard for the rest of it. "Ask and you shall receive." I learned to be more specific in the asking. That week, I needed to go to Tirana, the capitol, to get my money. I went by train, and it was a four-hour cold trip. Most Albanians read while traveling. I was reading the Roman's Road in the Albanian Bible and trying to practice reading it. There were eight of us in the train car together, and one of them asked me what book I was reading. I replied in Shqip: "Bibla, Fjala e Zotit" (The Bible, God's Word). They asked me where I was from, how many years had I studied Shqip because they couldn't believe that I knew it, and who taught me. I told them Jesus Christ gave me their language. Since they were interested in the book I was reading, I showed them the Roman's Road. One person left the train car because he didn't want to hear, but the others stayed as a captive audience. After reading and explaining the Gospel, several of them bowed their heads and prayed a sinner's prayer. Only the Lord knows who got saved that day, but they all heard for the first time how they can have eternal life.

The train would stop, and to my horror, some of the new believers would get off the train without a tract, a Bible, or even a contact.

We didn't have cell phones nor physical addresses. Churches were far and few between in those days. One of the best things that comforted me was that I knew that they who had truly believed had the Holy Spirit living and dwelling within them. *He* would never leave them nor forsake them!

Tell one experience about your early days in Albania.

Here's the story about how the Lord removed the Arab organization from the school-age orphanage and from Albania and saved many orphans!

Secret Meeting, 1997

Working with Maria, the preschool orphanage director, I was invited to many different functions. One week, an NGO (nongovernmental organization) named Red Barnett was holding a training session for the directors and some of the educators of the orphanages. It was at our preschool orphanage. All the directors in Shkoder attended plus the director over all the orphanages, Bepi. When he found out that I was an American, unbeknownst to me, he had hoped that I could help him with an urgent situation. He came for a visit to my house and stood outside asking me to please come to his house for a visit, to visit him and his family, and to discuss a very dangerous problem. He told me that I couldn't tell anybody because our lives could be in danger if the word got to the wrong people.

I brought Mirela, my assistant, with me to Bepi's home so that she could translate. She was learning English but didn't know it very well. We got past the formalities of a visit, and then I asked him what was so urgent. Before he went on, he looked us both square in the face and asked us to promise not to tell anybody in Albania about this secret meeting because we were all at risk of death if word got out to the wrong people.

He happily started telling us how that for the past four years, whenever Hope for the World (HFTW) came to Albania to help their government with the orphans here in Shkoder, he had seen a huge difference in them and the facilities. As he spoke, there was joy and peace pouring out of him.

"The facilities are much better because many changes and repairs have happened. They are painted and kept up. The children are certainly much happier, cleaner, and healthier than prior to HFTW's help," he said.

Mirela was translating for me because some of the words he was using I hadn't learned, and he was talking with so much passion that he spoke very quickly. He continued on telling us how that when he went up to the children to give them a hug before HFTW came, the children would throw up their arms over their heads and faces to protect them from being hit. Now, they run up to him and give him hugs and don't throw up their arms over their heads but throw them up to receive and give hugs with huge smiles on their faces instead of fear!

He sadly went on to say, "This is not the case at the school-age orphanage with the Arab 'humanitarian' organization. The children are not healthier nor cleaner. They cover their heads and faces with their arms to protect themselves from being beaten when approached to be given a hug!" He started getting very angry and dramatic as he stood up and started slinging his arms around in despair. His whole demeanor changed to that of an aggressive one. I didn't understand what he was verbally saying, but I knew that he was in desperation.

I prayed. Mirela stopped interpreting for me and explained it all after he calmed down.

While the drama went on, I prayed. Mirela finally explained the following to me. Bepi even drew me a diagram. This director is like a puppet whose hands are tied. He tried talking to the Albanian government, but they only laughed at him. The Arabs were using that orphanage as a front to hide their weapons for terrorism. They were forcing the children to learn the Koran and to pray five times a day after the Islamic faith. This was against the law. After communism fell, there was a law that stated you had religious freedom. There were some children who were Catholic, and they weren't allowed to read the Bible nor go to church but were forced to worship Allah. Whenever the nuns went to pick up those children to bring to church, the Arabs didn't allow them.

This "humanitarian" organization didn't do projects to help the facilities nor buy new clothes or things for the children. They circumcised the children at the orphanage as part of an Islamic religious ceremony. During the orphans' yearly summer vacation at the beach, they forced the girls to swim in the garbs (I don't know what you call them), all wrapped up from head to toe. Some of the girls were being raped. It was a terrible situation, and he was asking America for help.

I asked him how he thought I could help. He told me to tell the newspapers, radio, and even the president. He was really desperate, and it was written all over his face and being. He gave me a handwritten four-page letter with names, dates, and events so that I could send it to America and get help. Again, he reiterated how dangerous that letter was and to be very careful that nobody gets it. I felt like I was an actress in an action movie with spies, murderers, and terrorists. I was still taking in all the events of the past hour and a half. I took the letter and continued to pray. Before we left, I prayed out loud that our great God Almighty would take care of this situation and put it in his powerful hands. We said our goodbyes and left that exhausted despairing man with some hope that Christ was going to prevail over the enemies.

I remember walking away from that place with Mirela asking her if she could believe what he said. She really did as I did, too. Then, when we finally arrived at my house, we talked about how she was going to translate that letter. I gave her my Albanian/English and English/Albanian dictionaries so that she could work on that letter. We couldn't believe that this director was asking me, a simple teacher, to help move terrorists out of the orphanage and out of this country! I laughed at the Lord in disbelief that *he* gave me this mission. But Mirela and I knew what to do, pray! And we did.

Mirela used a flashlight whenever everybody in her family was sleeping and worked on translating that letter every night for the next week. It was done just in time for when our HFTW director,

Roger Mullins, came in the country. I was able to hand deliver it to him, and he said the same thing I did. "All we can do is pray." I left for America shortly after that incident and shared this situation with all our brothers and sisters in Christ, as an urgent prayer request. This was about the time the Lord gave me the mustard seed faith idea. I was in Georgia visiting Brother Roger and Cherie and gave Brother Roger a mustard seed which I had simply glued to a piece of paper with Matthew 17:20 typed on it. I told Brother Roger that we needed this much faith to move that Arab mountain out of the school-age orphanage. I received a phone call several months later from Brother Roger telling me that he had received a phone call from the Albanian government telling him that they kicked out the Arabs and that organization out of the orphanage and out of the country!

They proceeded to ask Roger if HFTW would consider moving in and helping them out just like we were doing in Tirana and Shkoder. Roger asked me if I would consider going there as well as to the preschool orphanage! I gladly praised the Lord and said *yes*! When I arrived in that orphanage in November of 1997, I found a Koran on each of the pillows of the 130 children's beds. Praise the Lord Jesus Christ who protects and answers prayers! Those Korans were eventually replaced with the Bible. Many of those children were saved over the years, and their lives forever changed for the good! I praise the Lord for HFTW and their sponsors' prayers.

Editor's note: I needed to insert a wonderful praise right here because it would not have been possible for us to take over that school-age orphanage if we were not able to provide $2,000 of help every month. We would have to execute a contract with the Ministry of Labor and Social Services in order for us to walk into that open door and bring the Gospel of peace and the love of Christ to those children. Roger and I happened to be going to a church in Fort Worth, Texas, for a revival meeting and were presenting Hope for the World on Sunday in the morning service.

It just so "happened" (or did it?) that our long-time friends and supporters, Carl and Vernice Howard, came up from San Antonio, Texas, to join us that day. To those who have read my previous book, you have read quite a bit about this family already. Roger made a plea that morning for prayer and for anyone who would help us to be able to get that orphanage under our wing and under God's protection. Well, much to our surprise, Brother Carl stood up and said, "You can tell them you'll have that $2,000 each month, Brother Roger, because I'm going to send it to you." Well, can you imagine how our hearts started beating fast and tears streaming down our faces? We had it! We knew Carl was going to keep his word because they had been a big part of our ministry for many years and were always faithful to all of their commitments. This was just the largest commitment we had ever seen anyone make! We were so blessed and were able to call our leaders in Albania and tell them to get the contract written, and we began then and there to be the spiritual leadership working in that orphanage with kids from the ages of seven to fourteen. We are still there today. Praise the Lord!

Now, back to the rest of Theresa's story.

What have you been doing there for all these years?

I worked with HFTW for five years hiring and training nationals to do my job. After the Lord blessed HFTW with three orphanages in Shkoder during those five years, the Lord had qualified Albanian workers in all three of those orphanages, and I literally had worked myself out of a job. That's what missionaries are supposed to do!

For the next ten years, the Lord had me sharing the glorious Gospel with Fredi and Prenda's family members in their many remote Alpine villages. I taught the Bible to the village women and children. As the children started getting saved and growing older, I trained them to teach the other children and gave them teaching materials so they could teach. I also helped with humanitarian aid whenever the Lord provided in addition to helping with our church in Shkoder.

Since 2011, I've been living in and shining Christ's light in Bajram Curri, helping our national missionaries, Pastor Astrit and Vjollca, with our church planting efforts in Tropoje and in Kosova.

You can see that when Theresa surrendered as a missionary, she *truly* surrendered! Her whole life has been there in Albania since 1995. She is a missionary of all missionaries! We are so happy that God allowed her to be the very first assignment we had in Albania.

Hope for the World Albania has been supporting Pastor Astrit Zefi (where Theresa is now involved) and this work in Tropoje ever since they began. We have been so blessed to watch it grow and see many, many come to know Christ. They are also involved in a wonderful program of feeding hungry children from the surrounding area.

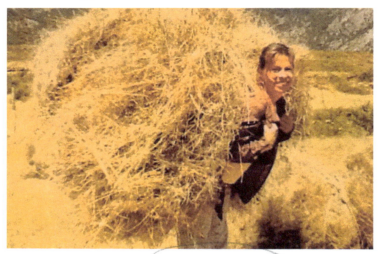

I loved this photo of Theresa. She Is a very hard working Missionary. She loves to help the people in all they are Doing, but I think this load was a little bigger than she Would have been carrying, More of a 'photo op'.

A Slumber Party to Remember

Since I have been talking about Theresa, it brought to mind another very special occasion that she and I were both involved in. I recall that we were in Albania during Easter season that year. It was April 15, 2001. This happened to be the very first Easter after our employee's, Prenda Zefi, mother had passed away on Christmas Day of 2000. It is always a very sad time for families to gather on special days like this without one of their loved ones, and in Albania, it is customary for the family to gather and to really sort of hold a special mourning and remembrance day. Well, Prenda and Fredi had been with us on Sunday at church in Shkodra, and since we had a couple of days yet before we had to make a move to another city, Prenda asked me if I might go with her to her sister Dava's home and spend the night with her and all of her sisters. Her sisters being Dava, Mrika, Dila, and Bardhja. All of them were already there together, and Prenda and I arrived late in the evening to spend the night in this tiny little apartment with just *one* bedroom. Theresa Weaver was there as well, and she was going to spend the night close by with another member of the family, if I remember correctly. Where were we all going to sleep in that little one-bedroom house? I had no idea!

When Prenda and I arrived at Dava's that night, she was cooking and getting ready to serve us a meal, which I enjoyed with them. Her apartment was very, very small, and I really wondered how we were all going to stay there. I believe there was another relative nearby, and a couple of the group went there to spend the night. I just remember how somber and sad everyone seemed to be. It is hard for me to not try to have fun with people when I get together in a group, especially a group of women. These ladies were strangers to me, except for Prenda and Dava. Really, I didn't know Dava very well at that point. I just knew that she had given her heart to Christ after Prenda had, and they were the only ones of the sisters who were saved at that time.

My poor attempt at speaking Shqip with them was really so funny it actually made them laugh, and then I would use Prenda as my interpreter and tell them funny things that would really get them laughing and enjoying our time together. It seemed that the more things we shared, the more fun it was, and the better we all got to know one another. I remember that Prenda's older sister, Mrika, sat near me and either held my hand or rubbed my arm or patted my hand the whole time and would not leave my side. And Dava was the busy one, in the kitchen and going about serving everyone. It made me think of the story of Mary and Martha in the Bible when Jesus came to visit. They were all so very respectful of me, I'm sure due to my age being close to their mother's. And they were interested in the fact that I was also bearing the testimony of a Christian. They had not seen many "senior citizen Christians" yet. This made them pretty interested in my life, I believe.

We had such a good time. We laughed, we cried, and we shared things about God with them. When it came time for us to go to our beds, I found out that about six of us were all going to sleep in the same one bedroom. It was filled with wall-to-wall beds. I had one single bed on one side of the room, and then there were other beds for the sisters to share beside me. I so wanted Prenda's three sisters who had not yet been saved to come to know Christ, so I decided to give them one illustration that I thought would help them know how simple it was to let Christ into their hearts. I got out of my bed and stood up and told them that to become a Christian was as simple as this. There was a door to the bedroom. I said, "I am going outside of that door and will knock on the door."

Prenda is, of course, translating this for them.

"I will represent Jesus knocking right now on your heart's door. He wants to come in, but he will not come in unless you invite him in." I said, "Now I am going outside this door and will knock. Someone, please come and open the door and invite me in."

I went outside the door. Mrika was near the door, and she opened it and asked me to come in. When I came in, I then shared that this is how easy it is to ask Jesus into your heart and life. He wants to come in, and he will live with you from then on, but you have to *personally* invite him into your heart and life. Ask him to come and be at home in your heart. With that, I just went to bed and said good night to them.

In the morning, before I was really very wide awake, I felt someone sit down on the edge of my bed and lean over and put her head on my shoulder. It was Bardhaj. She was crying. I asked Prenda to come and translate for me. Bardhaj wanted to open her heart's door to Christ that morning. Dila wanted me to know that she had opened her heart's door to Jesus and invited him into her life as her Savior. That same morning, I also learned that Mrika had done the very same thing the night before after they went to bed. I had heard them whispering with Prenda for a long time after I lay down. Of course, I did not understand anything they were saying but found out about it the next morning. That made all of the sisters now born-again believers! What an awesome time of rejoicing we had together with Theresa Weaver, the missionary who was working with us. She had been so instrumental in bringing the good news of the gospel to members of their families and even to them. We all shared together in a great day of rejoicing! That was a sleepover I will never forget as long as I live. I am happy to say that these ladies and their families have been growing in the Lord from that day on.

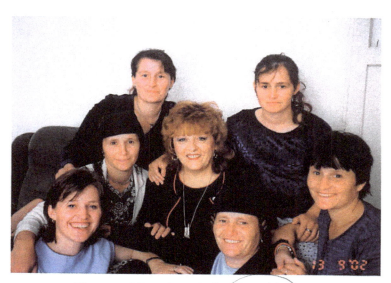

Cherie and Prenda and all of Prenda's sisters
What an awesome night we had I I love these Ladies so much.

Alketa: A First Employee

I am an Albanian girl, and I became a Christian in Albania in 1996, just a few short years after the communist regime ended in Albania. We were only open to the Gospel again beginning in 1992 in my country. After I was saved, it was my heart's desire to be able to share God's truth, love, and salvation with other people. I prayed that the Lord would put me in a place where I could talk about my Savior, Jesus Christ, and what he had done for me and for all people.

In December of 1997, I was asked by our missionary, Theresa Weaver, if I would be interested in working with Hope for the World in the orphanages in my hometown of Shkoder. I prayed about it and was so excited to work with the orphans.

I will never forget my first day. As I entered the building at the orphanage, I was surrounded by the children. Many of them were wondering why I was there. I told them that I was going to work for a Christian organization and that we were going to be there to love and care for them. At first, it was hard to see the pain and darkness in the hearts and eyes of many of the older children, as they had been through so much.

Over time, however, the Lord blessed Theresa and I with the ability to build great relationships with the children and staff which was made up of government workers who knew nothing about the God of the Bible. Through our daily serving and sharing the gospel, they were able to see the light and hope in us. They received the daily reminders from God's Word, love from us, and salvation through Jesus Christ. The children were eager to hear about a Savior who loved them and died for them. They loved knowing they had a heavenly father who cared for them and loved them, as most of them had no earthly father who did so. Some were not even living.

After a few months, God blessed me with the ability to lead one of the girls named Stela to pray and accept the Lord as her personal Savior. What an indescribable joy and blessing that was. I was so thankful to be used for the Lord's glory.

Working with Theresa Weaver through Hope for the World in the orphanages was one of the best experiences of my life. Having come to know Roger and Cherie Mullins was an amazing experience. The love and effort they have poured into Albania and the Lord's work there as a whole give us all an example that we can follow. I truly count myself blessed to call them my friends.

God blessed me tremendously as I was working there with HFTW. During the Kosovo crisis in my country when we were making special rescue camps for Kosovan refugees in my town of Shkoder, I came to know some wonderful American doctors. I volunteered to help them mainly with translating for them as they tried to help so many of the refugees there. They saw I had a real heart and talent for the medical field, and it was through this connection that I later got to go to America, to the State of Washington, and train for a profession in the medical field. I will never get over this wonderful opportunity.

While living there in Washington, God led me to a wonderful Christian man named Tom Carlson. We soon married and now have a beautiful family and are very happily serving the Lord. I cannot praise God enough for the blessings he has given to us.

I still look back to the day I found Christ, however, in Albania, just a few years after the doors of communism closed in my country. Then for the years I was able to learn through Theresa Weaver and others with Hope for the World to give my all to the Lord, I am so thankful. I appreciate Cherie giving me the chance to put my memories in her book. I hope if anyone is reading this who does not know Christ as Savior, you will come to him. You can find him if you seek him with your whole heart. I did, and he will never leave me nor forsake me.

In Christ alone,
"Keti"

Second Granddaughter

It was on June 13, 2000, that Kerri gave birth to their second daughter, Jacklyn Olivia Mullins. Yes, Tori now had a baby sister, and what a beautiful little girl she was! I am putting some photos of these two little girls in this book so you can see for yourself! Yes, Livi was so very beautiful; she could have been a wonderful poster baby for many baby products. My goodness, what a little doll she was! Her big sister loved her to death! They were so cute as Victoria would sit and hold Olivia on her lap. She was like a little mommy for sure.

I have mentioned a few times Wes and April Willett, who were Buddy and Kerri's best friends. Well, just three months before Olivia was born, they had their baby girl, Gracie. Yes! She was just three months old when Olivia was born, and wouldn't you know it, they became the very best friends from their beginning. They really did! Sixteen years later, and they are still very close friends. What a blessing!

Neena (Kerri's mother) worked so hard making some of the most gorgeous little frilly dresses you could ever imagine. The girls had matching dresses a lot of the time. Many of them were full-length, down to their little shoe tops, with many ruffles and tucks. And, of course, there were matching hats sometimes. They were so blessed to have this talented grandma doing all of this sewing for them. Kerri's mom and dad have always been such great helpers with the girls. They also were always a part of each move they made, and they made several. They would be on hand for the move and the interior decorating by making everything from window treatments to bedding, pillows, lampshades, upholstered furniture, you name it. Neena is so gifted in all of these things, and Papa has the patience of Job and knows how to salvage anything and completely make it over or help with all types of remodeling. Whatever Kerri could think up, her dad could help her put it together. Buddy took after his parents, his talents were not in any of those fields, although I will say that having Kerri's parents in their lives all these years has helped Buddy learn to be much more handy around the house. What he got from his family was mainly in the lines of music and ministry. I know that we always felt that Buddy was so blessed by marrying Kerri Anne King. He not only got her, but he got the greatest in-laws in the world, just as Cindy did when she married into the Howard family.

Well, now I've told you that our fourth grandchild had entered our world. Jacklyn Olivia. She has grown up through the years to be a very, very special young lady today. She is an excellent academic scholar. School has always been really easy for her, and she has excelled in all of her studies. She has loved her big sister and, of course, wanted to be a part of the same things Victoria was doing but was too young for a long time to really be able to be included when Victoria went off with her own friends. Livi has always seemed content to stay around the house. She's been a helper to her mom and probably a deeper thinker than some of us realized. She inherited the same talent for singing and playing instruments that her dad has. She also shares that same passion we saw in Buddy at her age.

Livi began very young exercising her musical abilities. In fact, she had her own part in one of our family recordings called "Wonderful Life" that included each one of the grandchildren. They each actually had a solo on the project. Her part was a little brief but very cute. When they sang the words "And if the devil doesn't like it he can sit on a tack," it was Livi's part to yell "ouch" right there. She always did it perfectly at home when we would practice, but she stubbornly refused to do it at the time we were recording. Everyone was coaxing her to do it, but she would shake her little head negatively and simply refuse. Well, we all took our time trying to get her to put her part in, but it was finally Poppy who had the magic touch and he sat down beside her on her stool, and soon she was in full cooperation and did it perfectly. It's so neat that we got to capture their voices at the time when she was three, Tori was seven, Austin was nine, and Brady was thirteen. That was their first family recording project. Then, a few years later, their voices were all heard again on our "Home for Christmas" project.

Now as I'm writing this, Olivia has just graduated from high school. The things she has been involved in at her school have been truly amazing. She has found two real great girls her age who are also very talented in music, both singing and playing guitar. They have formed their own little group and called themselves "SOL" which is made from their first initials, Savannah, Olivia, and Logan. They are serious about their music! They have connected with a wonderful songwriter who is a musician in their church and also a part of the Nashville music world. He has been mentoring them in their writing, arranging, playing, and singing skills. They have been invited to appear at a number of places in their beach-home area, around Santa Rosa Beach, Florida. The girls also use their talents in their churches and have led a number of praise and worship services during their sophomore year of high school.

Another hidden talent Livi had that we really didn't know about, until she agreed to play the role of Wednesday of *The Addams Family* in their high school musical, is acting. She was super in that comedic role and had some great solos that she did with perfection. As a result, she recently was awarded the "best actress of the year" award at her school's awards evening. So though we thought only Victoria was the actress, it now appears there are two of them!

Oh, it is so much fun having your grandkids entertain you! We are so very proud of all four of ours, and we are actually blessed to death!

A new church was launched in their town recently. Both Livi and Tori are a very active part of that new church plant. Livi has actually become the worship leader for the music in the church. She loves this dearly and does an amazing job with the Praise Band. Victoria has a role in assisting the pastor's wife in planning, organizing, and helping with small groups within the church. During the weekdays, they meet in people's homes, but on Sunday, they are in a local theater. The church has grown tremendously within the one year it has been going. I can't tell you what a blessing these girls are to us. God has been good, extremely good to us. And as I am finishing this book for publication, Victoria had been engaged, and she and Matthew Richard married each other on February 16, 2019. Matthew is also involved in ministry as an assistant pastor of the church in Florida. It is called "Impulse Church" and is growing weekly and reaching many souls for Christ.

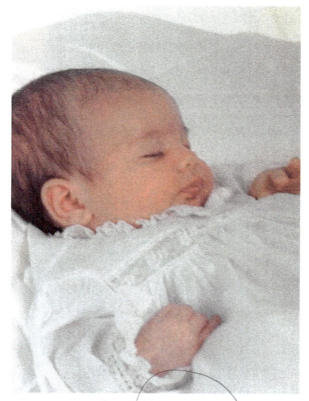

Second Granddaughter—Olivia
Beautiful little Livi—Born June 13, 2000
To our son, Buddy and wife, Kerri Mullins

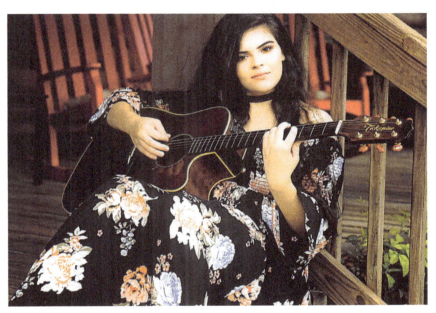

Second Granddaughter—Olivia
Senior Picture—She has a passion for music!
Is The Worship leader in her church

Marga: An Orphan's Story

I asked my friend, Marga, if she would mind telling you her life story as she was one of the first teenage orphan girls we came to know when we first went into Albania with Hope for the World. She had quite a life up until that time and has a very compelling story to share with you. At the end of her story, I will share with you something very, very exciting, so please read and feel her pain just knowing that you are not alone, as the Lord feels our pain and is our wonderful comforter. I hope you will be blessed by the story of Marga's life.

My life verse is Psalms 27:10: "When my mother and my father forsake me, the Lord will lift me up."

My name is Margarita Cyri, and I am from Albania. I came to America over a decade ago. Since then, I went to college and graduated with a broadcasting degree, found a job, and recently got married to the most amazing man! God has been so good to me. It wasn't easy to get to this point. Let me tell you what an amazing work my God has done in my life.

As a little baby, I was sent to the baby orphanage south of Albania in Vlora. I was able to live there for six years. During that time, being so young, I can't remember much of what happened. All I can remember was that one day, this beautiful lady came to see us and brought me a present of fruits and food. She smiled at me, and I smiled back at her. At that time, I was only three years old. That beautiful lady left, and I never saw her again. At the age of six, I was moved to the bigger kids' orphanage. Mind you, the atmosphere there wasn't that pleasant. That building was equipped to hold over one hundred kids at one time. The bedrooms were big. There were two floors with six bedrooms each, one floor for the boys and one floor for the girls. On one side, there were three bedrooms where we were separated by grades. Grades one through four were in one side of the floor, and grades five through eight were on the other side of the floor. One room held at least twenty to thirty kids. You do the math. At the age of eleven or so, we had to wash our clothes by hand. At that time, we had no washing machines and dryers. Talk about growing up fast! That was life at the orphanage.

From the time I set foot in that orphanage to the time I left, I had quite a life. Yes, there were some laughing moments, but for the most part, it wasn't a happy place. Ever since I was a child, I was made fun of. As a little girl, I used to be very quiet. That is one thing older girls and boys didn't like about me. I would get beaten up for being that way. Also, going to bed at night was mostly a nightmare more than anything else. I knew exactly what would happen. The older girls would come and wake some of us up and put us each in the bathroom stalls and touch us inappropriately. Oh, the nightmares were long. It seemed like it was going on forever. The next morning, we had to wake up early and walk to school. Sometimes, we would go to school with finger marks on our faces from being slapped so hard. The educators would see that, but what could they do? I dreaded every time I went to school. You could very easily tell the orphans from the children who had parents. All the orphans dressed alike. We had the same haircut. Just as if we didn't have enough abuse at the orphanage, it would still go on at school. The teachers had the liberty to call on you and even be physical with you if they saw fit. I hated it. All I kept saying was, "It's just not fair. What did we ever do to deserve something like this?"

When food or something else was stolen in the classrooms at school, guess who was blamed for it—the orphans. It is funny now, but it was not funny then. On the way to school and coming back, we used to pick up gum from the ground and put it in our mouths. Mind you, that gum had been stepped on by who knows whom, and it would end up in our mouths. For the most part, we would go hungry to school. We couldn't wait until school was done so we could walk back and eat. Bread was one of the many things that was filling to us. Growing up under communism wasn't fun at all. As orphans, we were hated because the mentality was that families would work so hard and we were eating the fruit of their labor. We were considered our dictator's children.

My country of Albania was under communism for five decades. Our dictator's name was Enver Hoxha. According to him, there was no God that existed in this world. Albania was a Christian country many years ago. History tells us that when the Turks came and took over our country over five hundred years ago, we became a Muslim nation. Later, Albania took over the Turks and defeated them which resulted in independence from the Turks. When our dictator, Enver Hoxha, took over the country, he decided that anything that had to do with God should be burned and wiped out from the earth. Thus, we became an atheist country. For years, we were taught evolution. We were told that we were created from monkeys and they would show the evolution of the monkey turning into a man. We didn't know any better.

Every year in the summer, we would go down south to the city of Vlora for vacation. We loved to go to the beach. One day, when we were at the beach, an older man came and started talking to me. I was only twelve years old. He noticed I had a problem with my eyes. He happened to be an eye doctor. The best part was that he said that he was my cousin. The longer we talked, the more he liked me. We even walked together with the other children up to the camp where we were all staying, and he wanted to take me home. That day was the happiest day of my life. I was going to go home with my cousin who happened to be an eye doctor, and I was going to be taken care of. Well, after going home with him, he took me to what he told me was my grandparents' house. What was going to be a two-week fun stay with them turned out to be barely a one-week stay. During that time, my "grandparents" told me how they named me and other things. To me, as a twelve-year-old girl, everything they said sounded so real. Little did I know that everything they were saying was a lie.

THE MAKING OF A WONDERFUL LIFE

One day, I was sitting with them to eat lunch, and at that time, I still didn't know how to eat meat with a fork and knife. So my twelve-year-old instinct was to dig my hand into the dish and put the meat in my mouth. That gesture didn't go over too well with my so-called grandparents. They were very upset. I couldn't believe it. They started to yell at me, and they didn't want anything to do with me anymore. All I could do was watch and listen until my so-called cousin, the eye doctor that I met at the beach, came to send me back to the camp with all the other orphans. I was very sad. I went to give my "grandparents" a hug, and they didn't accept that. All I could do was cry. The worst part was that once the word was spread at the camp in Vlora, I became the most disappointed child in that camp. I was ridiculed and had to hear it for what seemed the longest time ever. Even when we went back to the orphanage in Tirana after the vacation was over, I had to hear it again and again from everybody. All I could think of was "I'm such a disappointment." What hurt the most was the fact that this gentleman who posed as my cousin, and this elderly couple who posed as my real grandparents, lied to me. But what could I do? I had no support or anyone to say, "It's OK, it is not your fault."

At the age of thirteen, I was eligible to have eye surgery to fix my eyes. It was the scariest thing I had to go through. I was terrified. Sadly, the surgery made my problem worse rather than better. During the time at the hospital, I was by myself for the most part. The worst part was when I woke up from having the surgery, I was totally alone. I couldn't even get my own drink and ask for help because I was so out of it. As I was trying to get the drink on my own, one nice lady came and helped me. At that moment, all I could do was cry and cry and cry and say thank you to the lady that helped me.

At the age of fourteen, I and my fellow orphans the same age moved out of the orphanage to the tech schools that our government decided to move us to. I was lucky in the fact that I was kept in Tirana but very scared because I was moving out to be on my own. Fourteen years old, on my own, at the high school dorm, you can imagine the look on my face—*terrified*. When I moved to the tech school dorm, I hardly had any clothes to wear. I only had one change of clothes. I would wash them, and that's what I would wear. I was usually cold. I don't remember the first time I ever got to buy new clothes. My life at the tech school was a living hell. Whereas at the orphanage we were in a room with twenty to thirty kids, in the high school dorm, we had double that. The worst part was we had bunk beds, so you get the picture. Being a fourteen-year-old girl, and on my own, was such a nightmare. Numerous times I had guys making advances toward me. Nothing ever happened, but it damaged me enough, physically, emotionally, and mentally. One of the guys even hit me really hard because he could not stand the fact that I kept turning him down. The verbal, physical, mental, and emotional abuse went on in the high school itself also. I was nothing but a joke to my teachers.

Since the government couldn't do anything for us in the summers, they would take all of us boys and girls and put us on the same floor, and we were just left to fend for ourselves. Mind you, when it was hot in Tirana, that dorm would have all the rats and mice possibly everywhere you walked. They were in the kitchen, along the hallways, in the showers, and even in the toilets. It was the worst nightmare ever that I had to live with for the longest time. I and my fellow orphans my age or older had to live with this ordeal for years. Being alone and having nowhere to go was one of the hardest things anyone could live with.

Two years later, when I was sixteen, our government decided that this particular summer, we teenagers at the tech school would be sent to Durres, which is about an hour away from Tirana, for a two-month "vacation." We were all put in one big van and sent to our destination. The first thing we girls experienced was a guy coming out of nowhere, flashing his private parts before our eyes. We could just imagine what the rest of our stay would be like. While in Durres, it happened that a riot was going on. We found out that this riot was for the fall of communism and the rise of democracy. That was a very new thing for us. This was in the summer of 1991. I, along with some of my friends, decided to go and join in the riot. When we all approached the port on the Adriatic Sea, oh, the scene that was playing in front of our eyes, there were two huge boats packed with people wanting to flee Albania and go to Italy. While I was totally lost in that scene for a while, I turned around to find myself totally alone. My heart pounded with fear! I didn't know where to go or who to ask for help. It was total chaos. While I was walking back to see if I could find someone that I knew, I found myself being followed by a stranger. I just knew something bad was going to happen because I was totally alone and couldn't find anyone to help me. Even the ones I thought I could ask for help totally ignored me. The stranger that was following me finally approached me, put his arm around me, and said, "I'll help you." At that point, there was no way of going back. I was trapped and led to a bunker, and that's when the ordeal started.

What I had feared would happen to me did happen. That day, I was sexually abused by several guys. The ordeal went on for what seemed like an eternity. From the noon hours to midnight, I was being sexually abused. During that time, I feared the possibility of being sold as a prostitute in Italy. As if the sexual, physical, emotional, and mental abuse weren't bad enough, I had to deal with the possibility of being sold as a prostitute in a foreign country. I began to wish I had never been born. When the ordeal was over, I was brought back to the camp where all my fellow orphans were, and they could tell what had happened to me. On the way walking back, I had fallen, I don't know where, but maybe on a swampy area because I was totally soaked. I couldn't speak, and I couldn't think straight. The next morning, I had to go see a doctor. While he was examining me, he wasn't being gentle at all. I was bleeding and crying uncontrollably. He told my male educator who took me to the doctor that there was a possibility that I had gotten pregnant and the doctor instructed my male educator to have sex with me so he could "help" me "not be pregnant anymore." Mind you, the previous day and night I was already used and abused. Now, I had to go through it again, but this time with my male educator. Would this nightmare ever stop? I felt that I had to do what the doctor said, so I did. That night was the longest night ever, and, finally, I gave up and said, "It hurts a lot. I can't do this anymore." The male educator was very mad at me, but at this point, I didn't care, I was in such pain.

I now had to live with what had happened for the rest of my life. The verbal, emotional, and mental abuse also continued. At this point, I had lost all hope. About that time, rumors started about "foreigners" coming to Albania, especially to Tirana, spreading God's word to the Albanian people. At first, I thought, *What?* And then I thought, *I don't know who God is, but I know for sure that I need him!* I found out that a church opened, close to the high school dorm I was living in. Since it was in walking distance, I went over there. The blond-haired blue-eyed pastor and his wife approached me and welcomed me to the church. I thought, *Wow! This is great!* I sat down and was amazed at seeing this foreign guy talking in English and an Albanian girl translating his words. So amazing! For a moment, I forgot everything I had gone through and concentrated on what this pastor had to say about God. I was also thinking, *I wish I knew English so I could translate like this girl is doing.* At first, it seemed so hard, but the more I went to this church, the better I was getting with learning English. That is how I pretty much learned how to speak in English—the pastor preaching and the interpreter translating. By the way, this pastor and his wife were from Sweden, and the church I went to was called "Word of Life."

Even though I was going to church at that time, I was still living in that same high school dorm, and the abuse I suffered there hadn't completely stopped. One particular night, as I, along with a couple of girls and a forty-year-old lady, was walking back to the dorm after church, two big guys came up. One of them grabbed my arm and asked the lady if he could "have" me for the whole night. She said, "No!" He got so mad at her that he let go of my arm and kicked the lady really hard. I thought of all the abuse I had endured over the summer, and now I had to deal with this. Such fear came over me that this man was going to hurt me. I was terrified, but nothing happened. Now, at that time, I was still in the very beginning steps of getting used to knowing that there is a God in heaven that takes care of his children. He had certainly taken care of me and my friends that night. So we were all able to get back to the dorm safely, but, to be honest with you, I was still scared to death. While living at the high school dorm, I heard that a group from America called "Pro-Missions" had come to help the orphans in Tirana. I thought, *Now those kids don't have to worry about who will take care of them, and they don't have to worry about going through the same hell on earth that I had gone through.*

During that time, one of my orphan friends asked me if I could go with her to the orphanage and go to church with her. I accepted her invitation. Another girl also came along with us. The three of us went to the orphanage, and this white-haired guy came walking toward us and asked us if we wanted to go to church with him and his group. His name was John, and he had brought a group with him from England. We all went to church with John and his group. When church was over, he asked if we could join him and his group for lunch. At that time, John and his group were staying at the "Tag Center." Their mission work was building and renovating the orphanage. While having lunch, one of the members, named Neil, began talking to me. Thank God, at that point in time, I had learned to speak English. It wasn't perfect but enough to communicate back and forth. Neil expressed a desire to help me. Mind you, I was already out of the orphanage and living in the high school dorm. After that, Neil came to see me every time he came to Albania. This English group directed by John had returned and started working on repairing a vocational school building that was going to house teenagers aged fourteen to eighteen. Again, wow! This was one miracle after another for the younger orphan teens. It was so amazing to see God at work to provide a safe haven for these teens. To be honest with you, I was happy, but I was a little jealous, too. I wished I was one of them. Well, my wish came true! When the vocational center was finally finished, forty-six teenagers moved in there from the orphanage in Tirana and from the high school dorm. I was one of them! I was so happy. The Pro-Missions organization at that time had been in Albania for a number of years. They were actually partnering with Hope for the World.

It was during this time that I began thinking about what was going to happen to me after I finished high school. I had only one year left. I still struggled with insecurities and also got in trouble a lot. One day, I remember it very well, I was punished by being restricted to my room for two weeks. The only times I could leave my room would be when I went to eat or go to the bathroom. Not really caring about obeying the rules, I went out of my room to stand in the hallway.

A lady came walking toward me with two of my fellow orphans on each side and said, "Hi, my name is Jean. What is your name?"

I said, "Marga."

She said, "So nice to meet you." And then she gave me a hug and said that she loved me. At this point, I really didn't care anymore about what would happen to me. What I didn't know was that this new organization called Hope for the World was getting ready to take over the orphanages in Tirana, and Jean was going to be the missionary lady that would stay with us and work with Hope for the World.

At first, I didn't like Jean at all. I thought she was just like everybody else who had been in my life, and I didn't believe a word she said. Let me tell you, Hope for the World could not have come at a better time in my life. I was seventeen years old and almost finished with high school. I was so afraid that I would have to return to that tech school where I had lived for two years and nothing good had come out of that. When Jean and Hope for the World came to work with us orphans, I was lucky to have known enough English for Jean to offer me a job to work for her and the organization. At first, I didn't think it was a good idea because of my past, but when I saw that Jean had a reason for asking me to work for her, I said, "Yes." Let me tell you, it was the best decision I ever made.

While all the other teenagers would go to school, I was put to work as an interpreter for Jean and Hope for the World. Did I still struggle with my English? Of course, I was still learning at that time. Just when I thought I was getting used to translating for Jean and the different groups that would come, here comes this well-dressed man, smelling good, gold chain around his neck, and gold bracelet on his wrist walking toward me all serious and tall. All I could think was, *Oh, my. I'll be translating for this man? I am in big trouble!* Mind you, I was only in my late teens. He told me his name was Roger Mullins. Then here comes this dolled-up lady following Roger and gives me a hug and says, "Oh, you will do OK. You will be fine. You can do it!" Her name was Cherie Mullins, and, to my shock, I didn't know she was his wife. But she was. This wonderful dolled-up lady helped me get over the fears I had in translating for her husband. She was good at putting me at ease. From then on, I was in good hands. While I was working as a translator, the missionary lady, Jean Williams, started to really see that I needed love and care. It's like she knew that I had gone through some hardships in life. She didn't know yet what had happened to me. Yet it didn't stop her from wanting to give me the love and care she thought I needed. She was one of those rare persons, and Hope for the World couldn't have asked for a better one than Jean.

While she was busy loving us and being there for us in Albania, at the same time, there was a wonderful couple in McDonough, Georgia, who were busy providing for us both physically and spiritually. One day, on a Sunday morning, I began wondering if I had ever truly gotten saved. To myself, I was thinking that since the pastor had laid his hands on my forehead and prayed for me, I had gotten saved. But I wasn't living like a saved child of God. I was still doing the same things, and even worse things, in my life that I am certainly not proud of, and I wasn't repenting of them. One particular day, Jean asked me what was wrong. I told her about what was bothering me and if she could please lead me to Christ. She was more than willing to do that. She took her Bible in English, and I got mine in Albanian, and she walked me through on how to get saved. That day, it was in February 1996, I received Jesus Christ as my Lord and Savior in my heart and in my life. I was so happy. I couldn't wait to tell everyone else that I was saved. I was the happiest girl in the whole wide world. At that time, I had already worked some for Hope for the World, and I was able to work for that organization for eight years.

During those years, I met many wonderful people who had been supporting the ministry. The best part of my work was when the sponsors from America would send money to their child in Tirana for their birthday. Oh, you should have seen those faces every time I would come and take them out so they could buy their birthday gifts and later that day we would go to the Stephen Center and eat pizza. While I was working with Hope for the World, the Lord was able to use me at church, too. Remember when I said that I'd love to be able to translate someday at church? Well, eventually, I was able to do that. The Lord was so good to me and used me in each and every way possible that he saw it fit. I was able to go to the villages and help my pastor with translating the messages. I was also able to lead the singing at church and in the villages where we ministered. I also helped with translating for the Kosovo people during their three months' war of independence from Serbia. During my eight years of working for Hope for the World in Albania, God used me in many different directions. My dreams had come true. What an amazing God he is! Thank the Lord for his many miracles in my life. God Bless you.

Editor's note: Actually, this is going to be quite a lengthy note concerning Marga, but it has to be told, so stay with me for "the rest of the story" as the late and great Paul Harvey would always say.

There comes a time in the lives of most foreign missionaries, when they return home for many different reasons, and that time had come for our friend, Jean Williams. She was going to leave Albania and return to her home in Ohio, but she had also made provisions and arrangements to get Marga enrolled in Pensacola Christian College in Florida. So they both came to America, and Marga was miraculously accepted as a student at PCC. She worked very hard all of the years of her education on campus. She was helped financially by various individuals and churches that permitted her to complete her education there and receive her BA in Broadcasting. During those years in college, she would sometimes come to our home on holidays and various vacation times, but mainly she stayed right there at the college and worked in order to defray her expenses.

After graduation, she moved to Ohio with Jean. She was in her late twenties by that time. She was having to go through many trials and tribulations with getting her green card so she could be gainfully employed, etc., and she was unable to fly because her visa had expired, so we didn't get to see her much at all for a long period of time.

Then, in late summer or early fall of 2014, she contacted us and let us know that she could fly again and wondered if she could come for a visit.

We were thrilled and said, "Yes, and why don't you come to be our special guest and give your testimony on Hope for the World Sunday at our church in October?"

So, she did! She hadn't changed, was just a little older, but the same live wire and ball of sunshine she had always been. She came in telling us that she really hoped that God would give her a wonderful southern Christian husband, and we were teasing her and laughing with her concerning this. She was thirty-eight years of age by now. Well, what we thought was joking, God heard as her heart's desire. She gave her testimony on Sunday morning, and it was so very touching, and she was "stunningly gorgeous" as she stood up there on the platform and just glowed with the love of Jesus. One of our most eligible bachelor friends was there that morning. He is especially close to us as he is a wonderful musician and he and I had played at church together on piano and organ and enjoyed it so very much. His name is Tony Waters. Well, it was actually him who had used those words "stunningly gorgeous" when talking about her to another mutual friend at church. The word got to me through that friend, and I was just happening to be chatting with Tony the next couple of days and he asked about Marga. I asked him if he would like to meet her personally. Well, he didn't hesitate to say yes, so we arranged for them to meet after prayer meeting that coming Wednesday. One thing that was so special about this is that both of them had always prayed for just the right soul mate, and neither of them wanted to marry someone who had been married before, but their chances were really getting very slim since they had already been in their adult years for a while.

Can I just bring this wonderful love story to a quick close by saying that it was truly a match made in heaven for those two? That was October, and by December, just before Christmas, they were united in marriage at our church. They are so happy! God truly has blessed Marga with a wonderful, loving, caring husband who can provide for her the rest of her life. They are members of our church and are a great blessing to all who know them.

I want to go right from this wonderful miracle about Marga to another one that took place in connection with some of our Albanian young people. I have asked Viola Demcellari to write about this in her own words. I believe you'll be blessed by her story.

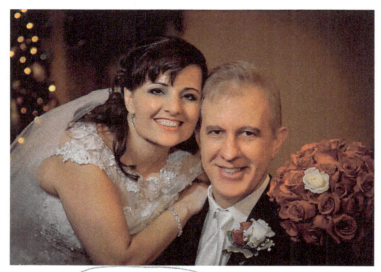

Marga and Tony Waters were married at Glen Haven Baptist Church, McDonough, GA Dec. 2014. Everyone was so happy for them.

Viola's Amazing Blessing

It all started with the Melville family visiting Albania on a mission trip with Hope for the World. They were sent from Harvest Baptist Church in Monroe, Georgia. They were called "The Light Ministries" and conducted puppet shows and songs and activities for the children in the orphanages and other places. Jerry, Ann, Melissa, Jessica, and Bethany Melville all came to Albania one summer, and a group of youth from New Hope Baptist Church in Tirana, Albania, accompanied them to interpret their puppet shows into Albanian. I was with that group of young people, and we visited the kids in the orphanage where shows were conducted for them as well as at New Hope Baptist church and the community.

One particular young man from New Hope Baptist approached Jerry and asked if it would be possible for him to study in the United States, as he was ready for college at that time. Jerry took that to heart, and upon returning to Monroe, Georgia, he shared the burden at church where a couple (Harold and Sheila Henson) took an interest in this matter. Due to some personal connections, they asked Mr. Herbert A. Mullenix, a trustee and member of the Board of Directors of Reinhardt College in Welaska, Georgia, if he could help. Mr. Mullenix had helped several students attend Reinhardt College (now Reinhardt University), and he agreed to sponsor this young man from Albania.

When The Melvilles notified the young man via Pastor David Young, the American pastor of New Hope Baptist Church in Tirana, that he could now attend Reinhardt, the young man had just heard from his application for a medical school in Albania where he had been accepted. He therefore had to make a choice, and he chose to stay in Albania and attend the medical school.

But now, there was an available scholarship fully paid for someone to attend Reinhardt, and Pastor David Young approached my dad to see if I was interested. I had at the time applied to universities in Albania and abroad and was awaiting entry testing to occur. We discussed this, and together we agreed Reinhardt would be a great opportunity for me. We also knew that the headquarters of Hope for the World Albania with our director, Roger Mullins, was also located within a couple of hours from this college. My parents also found some comfort in knowing that they were close by as they were in constant contact with the Mullins.

I had to get an English test done (called TOEFL), and once I was able to pass that, I started my application for Reinhardt. All of this had to happen quickly in order for me to be able to make the enrollment for that semester of college.

I arrived in the States in August of 1998 and stayed with the Melville family for a few nights and then was taken to Reinhardt campus for the start of school. They had planned a lovely reception at their church (Harvest Baptist of Monroe, Georgia), and I was presented with many nice and useful gifts which I would need for my dorm room. These included bedding, a lamp, toiletries, etc. This all turned out very, very handy as I came to America with just one suitcase of clothing.

The Melvilles' church family at Harvest Baptist also provided a van to come pick me up every weekend and drive me from Waleska to Monroe (a two-hour drive) so I could be with them and wouldn't be by myself for the first two years. They were like a second family to me, and I will be forever grateful.

During my third year at Reinhardt, Roger Mullins of Hope for the World, who of course knew me and my family as my dad worked for Hope for the World in Albania, approached me to find out how I had come to attend Reinhardt and was interested in bringing another young man from Albania, Alton Brinja, on the same scholarship. I spoke to Mr. Mullenix, and he agreed to sponsor another student from Albania, and Alton started attending. He also completed his education there at Reinhardt in four years, according to schedule.

Through the help of HFTW, my dad was able to visit the States and visit me on campus in my third year at Reinhardt. He could see where I had lived for a few years now. It was a very sweet and emotional moment when my dad arrived on campus. I didn't have a car or other means of transportation, so Brother Roger drove my dad up there. We then went for lunch, I believe. It was a fun day. We then attended the HFTW annual banquet in Florida afterward so I had the opportunity to visit there as well. It was our first time ever to go to Florida.

On my fourth and final year at Reinhardt, I approached Mr. Mullenix to see if my brother, Andi, could also be a beneficiary of his scholarship. Mr. Mullenix agreed as he was quite pleased that I was graduating with honors (cum laude) from Reinhardt and had been on the dean's list while in school. I graduated in May of 2002.

Andi started attending Reinhardt in August 2002. He had quite a list of accomplishments during his years there. He was the treasurer and later the president of RAMS (Reinhardt Association of Multicultural Students) during which time they had a project to enrich the school library with international writers and works based on the international background of students. Currently, the library has over one hundred books, including thirty Albanian books (in English). Andi was also the vice president of the Model of United Nations Reinhardt Association (MUNRA). For the first time in the school's history, they were able to represent the college in the prestigious Model of the United Nations held in the UN headquarters in New York City in March of 2005. He was a member of the student senate, a resident assistant in the school dorms, and Reinhardt captain under the admissions office to promote the university to prospective students. For that reason, he was also selected as a role model and pictured on the brochures of the university. He was vice president of the student government, chairman of the judicial council, and member of the Alpha Chi Honor society recognizing the top tenth percentile of students based on overall academic performance. He was also a member of Sigma Beta Delta, the Business Honor

Society recognizing the top tenth percentile of business students in academic performance.

Andi also graduated with honors of magna cum laude with a GPA of 3.7 and received his Bachelor of Science in Business Administration degree. He was selected in the 2006 edition of Who's Who among American Colleges and Universities and then in the 2007 edition for Young Professionals in America.

Mr. Mullenix passed away in 2005 while Andi was in his third year of college. The Mullenix scholarship ended for him, but because he was an excellent student and very involved, the school gave him a little grant.

We will forever be indebted to God for allowing this wonderful thing to happen for us. We do not take this for granted but count it as a miracle. We are also so grateful to Mr. Mullenix and his foundation for providing these scholarships for three Albanian students. The education was invaluable to us and has provided us with wonderful positive influences in our lives and enabled us to secure good jobs. Andi and I are both living in Canada now. I am married to a wonderful Albanian man whom I knew in Albania, and we have two children. We continue to stay well informed and connected with Hope for the World and even do some translating for them from time to time between my father, Perparim Demcellari, and Brother Roger Mullins. To God be the glory for the great things he has done for me and our family.

Editor's note: I am so very happy that Viola and Andi were able to avail themselves of this opportunity. They were amazing students, as you can tell from reading their accomplishments, and are both a real credit to their country of Albania and to their parents. We are so very thankful that the Lord chose to put the Demcellari family in our ministry in 1999. Perparim and Aferdita have both been great friends and wonderful parents to their children and grandparents to their grandchildren. They are both spiritual role models to the young people in the orphanages and at our Hope Center as well as in their church. Our God goes ahead of us and plans the very best people and has them all ready for the job to which he later calls them. We have truly seen this not only in the Demcellari family but also in the lives of the wonderful staff members He has provided for us from the national Albanians from the very beginning of our ministry. We cannot praise him enough.

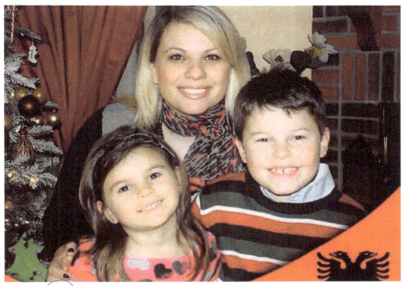

Viola and her two beautiful children. They live in Canada.

Andi Demcellari

And do not forget to do good and to share with others, for with such sacrifices God is pleased. (Hebrews 13:16)

When I first encountered the work of Hope for the World Albania, I could not fully comprehend the situation in Albania as I was only ten years old (in 1994) but old enough to understand that my country was going through many difficult moments. Despite not being an orphan myself, I was able to see firsthand the misery of living and spiritual conditions of the orphans in the "Zyber Hallulli" orphanage in Tirane, Albania. However, what I have as a vivid memory from that time is the joyous atmosphere and the love HFTW missionaries brought to kids in that orphanage.

Eight years later (2002), I was given the wonderful opportunity to study in the United States. That opportunity came from The Herbert Mullenix Scholarship Fund at Reinhardt College (now University) in Waleska, Georgia. By far, it is one of the milestones that has changed the course of my life ever since. With opportunity there was excitement but also a lot of fear of the unknown as I was only eighteen and never before had I lived by myself or been an ocean away from my parents. As I landed at the Atlanta Airport, I remember that I was scared. Now I was on my own, I thought. I had to figure out how to get to school. As I walked into the main terminal to pick up my luggage, I saw a familiar face. There was Roger Mullins with a big smile which was the best welcome I could have hoped for.

That day, he drove me to Reinhardt College. Patiently waiting for me to finish my check-in and registration, we went to lunch and then shopping to make sure that I had everything I needed. At the end of that first day, I was no longer scared but convinced that God will always make a way. From that moment on, I spent many weekends and holidays at Roger and Cherie's home in McDonough, Georgia. They made sure I had a home away from home.

During the years that followed, I gave it my best shot at being successful academically and also by getting involved in many student activities and organizations. It was the spiritual peace that I had that made it all possible. I was no longer feeling like an "outsider," and Georgia became my new home, and this is thanks to Roger and Cherie.

I graduated from Reinhardt in 2006 with honors of magna cum laude and had achieved a lot in my academics. I also served as vice president of the student government and president of the multicultural association, but now it was time to face the real working life. It was through the help of Roger and Cherie that I got an interview with a local businessman and was offered a job. After finishing college and getting some work experience, I decided to go back to Albania and work on my career there. Now, I live in London, Ontario, Canada. Many times, I look back and think, *How did I get this far?* One thing is for sure, without the help of people in my life, I would have never made it. Two of those people are Roger and Cherie Mullins who have always been good to me, and I am sure God is pleased

Andi Demcellari

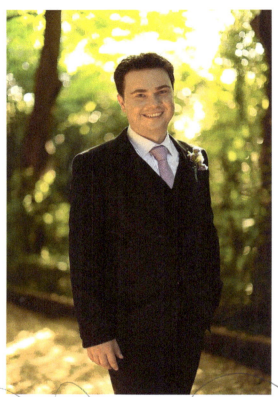

Viola and Andi are the children of our In-country President Perparim and his Wife, Aferdita. A wonderful family.

Etleva's Miracle

Our God is in heaven; he does whatever pleases Him. (Psalms 115:3)

Editor's note: This is another unbelievable miracle that was experienced during our early ministry years in Albania. Etleva tells it in her own words.

People: You cannot walk! Where ss your *Lord*? You will not walk!
Me: I will walk! I will walk!
God in me: Walk with Jesus precious child of mine! Walk with Jesus!

"Sometimes you will never know the true value of a moment until it becomes a memory." Here I am now, trying to put memories to words, to give memories colors, to give memories wings so they can fly around the world.

It all started the first week of April 2002. That week would mark the beginning of a new journey, an unexpected turn for my life, for my family's life. What occurred on that week would allow me to know God in ways that I would have never known if that did not happen. From 2002 to 2008, my God, in his sovereignty and for his glory, allowed pain, swellings, casts, crutches, wheelchairs, canes, stitches, surgeries, hospitals, physical therapy units, medical clinics, doctors, nurses, and therapists to be part of my daily life.

On the morning of April 1, 2002, I went to work and started discipleship training with one of the children from the orphanage where I worked. His name was Paolo. We finished the discipleship on James 4:13–17, and while going down the stairs, Paolo asked me: "Are you coming to pick me up to go shopping for my birthday?" Shopping for new clothes with the generous gifts from faithful sponsors of Hope for the World was a joyous and long-awaited moment for the children.

My response was: "Yes, yes, sure!" As quick as I said yes, that quick I took those words back, knowing that now was the exact moment to put into practice what we taught that day in discipleship. "Well, Paolo, we learned today that we should say 'Lord willing,' because now we are going down the stairs and I might hurt my feet, but I say to you that, Lord willing, I will come and pick you up, and we will go shopping for your birthday." On the afternoon of the same day, I went to play volleyball with my church group, and I hurt my ankle; a jump in the net, falling on somebody's foot, and then a twist. Ouch!

The long and painful, but joyous, journey had just begun! *Painfully dark*, still there is a light that lightens my path. *Painfully hard*, yet nothing is impossible for the Giver of Life. *Painfully hopeless*, till I lifted my eyes to the cross and to my Christ.

Without even knowing, I had just started an unexpected journey, of almost seven years, filled with medical problems. I went to my hometown hospital where the diagnosis was "torn ligaments." They put my foot in a half cast and said come back in two weeks. Words cannot express the pain I was in whenever I had to use crutches. In my mind I said, *OK, God knows what he is doing, I will make the most out of my time, so let's start to memorize the book of James.*

Two weeks passed by, so I went back to the doctor to get the cast off. When he took the cast off, all I could see was a very, very purple foot, all swollen up, and I could not move my toes at all.

The doctor said this: "Now it is fine. Just go on and walk."

I replied to him, "But I cannot move my foot. I cannot put it down. I cannot put weight on it. I am in excruciating pain."

Then he jumped on my foot saying, "There, you are just fine, just get up and walk."

In my mind, I was like, *Well, he is the doctor, he knows better than me, so I will endure the pain and walk.* Weeks went by and my foot was even more swollen, and by mid-June, my foot was as cold as ice.

One day, the missionary of the church where I was a member, Mr. David Hosaflook, came to visit me at my home. When he saw my foot, he said that something should be done, that maybe I needed to go for a visit to a clinic in Tirana, the capital city of Albania, and he suggested a Korean clinic there. He drove my brother and me there. Once we got there, I explained in detail everything. The first thing the doctor said was: "The doctor's advice to walk on your foot has done more harm than help. We will put your foot in a cast again for two weeks. If nothing changes, you have to go out of Albania, because that means you need more specialized help." Two weeks went by again, I went back to the Korean clinic, and took off the cast. The foot was even worse, more purple, more swollen, no mobility at all. Now what? Where do I go from here? What can I do? To what country could I go without a visa? Which hospital? How do we find the doctor? Where can we stay once we get there? The doctors were clear that in Albania, I could not get the help that I needed.

Days went by, days became weeks, the church where I was a member was praying for a solution, my family and me as well. My mother, my sister, my two brothers, and my older nephew were all believers at that time. They decided to fast every week, until God will open the doors that he wanted to. Well, after a couple of weeks, the answer came. The missionary of our church, David, had talked with a doctor at a hospital in Istanbul, Turkey, about my medical problems, and they had agreed to look at my case. We had another missionary couple, Pam and Keith Zellmer, that God used to bless us in finding a place to stay.

In the meantime, my father was working in Italy to help my family out. In our family of seven, I was the only other one working at that time. We talked with him and decided that my younger brother and I should go ahead and go to the hospital in Turkey and we would use all his savings if it was needed. The Hosaflooks loaned us their credit card so we could easily pay the medical bills, and my dad would reimburse them, which was easier than having him send the money to Turkey. "For my thoughts are not your thoughts, nor are your ways my ways, declares the Lord" (Isaiah 55:8).

My brother and I started a four-month-long journey, thinking that it would be a two-week one. We arrived in Istanbul in July 2002. David and Lucinda Williams opened the door of their house and their comforting arms to us. Their unconditional love for my brother and me was so obvious and still is. The day after we arrived in Istanbul, we went to the hospital, and yet another unexpected surprise. *News* from the first doctor's visit! I had acquired a disease because of my injury. Now I had a new problem, reflex sympathetic dystrophy (RSD). On that same day, I had a surgical procedure to put a tube in for the medication during therapy. I had therapy and went back to the Williams' house. At that time, I can tell you that I did not comprehend what was in store for me. I started therapy five times a week. Weeks passed by, and because I had not walked for months, the bones had started to show huge signs of gangrene. The doctor came and said, "If this continues with this speed, we might end up cutting your foot off." (Yeah, he said it like he was saying, "We might end up pulling your tooth out"). In the meantime, I started to have stomach problems, and while in Turkey, I ended up losing around thirty pounds and developed stomach ulcers.

Weeks went by with no improvement. One of the doctors at the hospital called my brother and me to his office and proposed to take out the sympathetic nerve, because they were thinking that this would help me start to walk.

I said, "I need some days to think before I decide." We went back to the Williams' and shared with them what the doctors just said. David found a lot of materials on that. I read all of it, and what always would go through my mind was: *Why should I accept to take out of my body forever something good and necessary that God created me with?* It turned out that, thank God, this was the best decision ever, because none of the doctors would have accepted to work with my case if I did have the sympathetic nerve removed.

Other weeks went by, and thankfully some improvement started to show up. The swelling went almost completely down, and I could bear some weight on it and finally start to take some steps after five long months. By November, I could walk, slowly, but at least I was walking. After meeting with the doctors, they told me, "This is as far as we can help you since this disease is new to us."

I went back to Albania, walking, praise God, with a disease in my foot and ulcers in my stomach. Three weeks after I got back to Albania, my foot got worse than it had ever been. The swelling went up to my knee now, and again I could not walk. In the beginning of December, brother Roger Mullins from Hope for the World, the foundation for which I was working, came to pay me a visit. I will never ever forget his tears, his loving kindness toward my sickness, my trial. "You are coming to the States," he said. "If you stay here, you will die." And that is what the doctors said when I went to the States.

Missionary David Hosaflook was able to find a doctor for my disease in South Carolina, and he and Roger and Cherie Mullins also got all the necessary paperwork for my visa.

My father's savings from Italy were gone in four months for surgeries, physical therapy, and food in Istanbul. I had on one hand my brother, ready to go to war to pay for my medical bills, and my family, ready to sell our house, but on the other hand, God was working graciously in the Mullins' hearts and hundreds of other people's hearts to support my new medical journey to the United States.

> When the misery of the sinful self drew me to You,
> I cried out "I am blessed, I am blessed."
> When your mercies cast away my blindness
> I shouted out "Glory to the 'I Am'."

How can I even think that I can sum up five years in the United States in a few pages? How can I do justice to thousands of people who have been enormous blessings and a vital part in my "lonely" journey? The Mullins raising funds for the medical bills. *(Editor's note: Our friends, Carl and Vernice Howard, from San Antonio, Texas, gave their credit card information to her specialist's office and told him to put her bills on their credit card.)* Hope for the World continued sending the check for my salary every month, and a lot of times, even more would come. The church body of Grace Bible Church, and all the members being involved in different ways, through prayers, driving me to and from doctor's appointments, physical therapy, and opening the door of their homes to host me. Then I am so thankful to Dr. Hess, Dr. Dunn, and Dr. Hobbs, for their services, appointments, and surgeries free of charge as well as the St. Francis Hospital in Greenville, South Carolina, for allowing all my multiple tests, surgeries, inpatient staying at the hospital, and physical therapy completely free of charge because I came from a third-world country and had a very low income.

The first time I stayed in the United States for one year during which time I started to walk again. The swelling was gone and also my stomach ulcers. Hence, I decided to go back to Albania. I was better. I could walk, why did I need to stay in the United States? Apart from all of this, the RSD doctor was not that sure, but my one-year visa was expiring, so I came back to Albania in January of 2004.

Within two weeks after I came back from the States, the disease went into both of my legs. My legs were swollen all the way up to the knees. We wrote to the doctor, and he said that I should immediately get back to the States because there was nothing he could do for me in Albania.

God was so gracious to work in people's hearts. Senator Jim DeMint was very kind to take time and write a letter to the American Embassy in Albania; God worked in the heart of the officials of the embassy, and I got the visa in two days, which in itself is a miracle. After four weeks of being back in Albania, I went back to the United States in a wheelchair. Being in a wheelchair was so very hard for me. I had to teach myself to not even think of it, even though I was wheelchair bound for two years. Physical pain was so much a part of me that I completely forgot how it was to be pain-free. After two years in a wheelchair, I was able to start to use a walker and afterward a four-prong cane. In 2008, the God of miracles, in his timing, answered our prayers. In that year, I started to walk on my feet, no walkers, no canes. Months went by, and the God of miracles did what the doctors did not ever foresee, I started to "run" on a treadmill!

In May of 2008, I started fasting and praying every Monday about the will of God for me. Did he want me in the United States, or did he want me to live in Albania and serve him here? After several weeks, answers started to come. In my head, I would ask myself these questions. *Why did you come to the States? To get better! Are you better? Yes! Do you see any open door from God or a reason that he wants you here? No!* Then, why do you wait? *Do you want that God should write it to you on a blimp?* "Etleva, I want you back in Albania." *No!* Then, go back, I will be with you! Hence, after almost five years in the States, I went back to my beloved country with a thankful heart and plenty of sweet memories but also difficult, painful memories as well, but I was now "running" for the miracle of my storm was over!

"Hallelujah to my Yahweh Shalom. Hallelujah to my Yahweh Jireh," is the melody of my heart for the lame sheep can run.

Hallelujah to my Yahweh Rapha. Hallelujah to my Yahweh Raah is the melody of my heart

(*Editor's note:* Let me say that Etleva was used mightily of the Lord while she was here in the States. She came several times to give her testimony at various programs where Roger and I were presenting our ministry of Hope for the World Albania. She would sometimes come and stay a few days with us, and we would enjoy shopping for some nice new fashions for her. We loved having her here. I remember how my youngest granddaughter, Olivia, loved Etleva. She was a blessing to everyone who met her. Many people still ask me about Etleva from time to time. When she began working on our staff in Albania, before her accident, she had finished college and had her degree in law, but there were very few opportunities for work in Albania at that time, and many well-educated people found it impossible to find a job in the field of their training. After all, it had not been much more than ten years since the fall of communism in their country. I remember that while Etleva was here in America, she was very busy writing articles for various publications in Albania having to do with extremely contemporary subjects related to business, etc. She kept abreast of all that was going on in her country. We are happy to report that since going back to Albania, she has a wonderful job in her field, and, in fact, just this past year, she received a very nice promotion. She was even sent to Israel representing professional women of Albania. God has blessed her, and she is physically fit and even able to wear very stylish heels today as you will see in the photos we are including. We love this lady, and I appreciate so much her sharing her story with us in my book.)

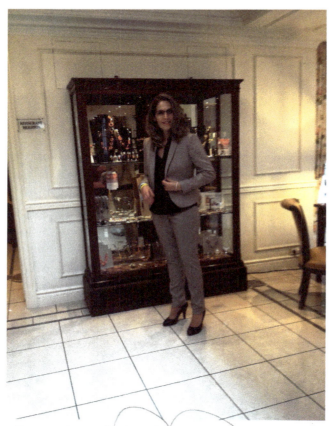

Recent photo of Etleva showing how normal her feet
And legs are now... A real Miracle!

Mentoring at Home

While our ministry is centered on and around Albanian orphans, and we spend part of our time traveling back and forth to Albania, the majority of our ministry happens here in America where we travel from church to church presenting our ministry. It is through the churches that we have been supported both personally and also on the field in Albania. Our own personal support comes from churches and also some individuals who we have continued to call our "Torchbearers" as that is what we called them during our evangelism years. They have been there holding the torch for us so we can see our way. Until you have been in full-time ministry that is fully funded by the gifts of God's people, you cannot imagine how important it is to have a support base. Our base consists of churches and Christian friends who care about our work, care for us personally, and are willing to give sacrificially to keep the work going that is reaching orphans, widows, and other souls in Albania. We are so grateful for each one who is a part of our ministry and has stuck with us for many, many years.

However, besides going from church to church, and doing our office work connected with Hope for the World throughout the years, God has at various times placed another special calling on our lives. In other books I have written, I have touched on this a little bit, how we have taken young men in to live in our home who have come from very troubled backgrounds or have been in some sort of addiction and have not fared very well by going the route of rehab facilities. For some reason, God has burdened us for these young men, and at different stages in our lives, we were impressed to reach out and help someone who really needed help. This was the case right in the midst of our first ten years of our mission work in Albania.

We had been to another country not far from America where we had ministered for many years at various times, in the islands of the Bahamas. There we had met and come to know and love many, many of the people who lived there. One particular family had a son who had been raised in church, had professed to be a Christian, but had gone the way, you might say, of the prodigal son. He had gotten himself entangled deeply in the things of this world, and it led to his parents trying many, many different Christian rehab centers in many, many places. He had started this pattern of life at about age sixteen, and at this particular time, when we became aware of how serious it was, he was approximately twenty-eight years old. We knew him personally, and when we were there visiting in his hometown, which is on an island, we spent some time with him. He had been back home for a while, and during that time, he had seemed to have another serious encounter with the Lord in his life. As a matter of fact, he told us that he really and truly had recently become a born-again Christian and he knew it for certain, and he wanted to do something for the Lord with his life.

His problem was that he had blown it, you might say, with the people where he lived, as far as trust or confidence. No one would probably believe him and his recent determination to straighten up and live for the Lord. It was going to be very difficult to make them believe that he was truly converted, and so, naturally, he didn't have much hope that anyone there where he lived would try to employ him or even trust him around their own young people. He had spent some time in a jail on a neighboring island and had recently been released, and it was just a very, very dark time in his life, and he needed help.

Roger and I talked about it, and we were there in the Bahamas for another week or so ministering in the church. We felt that the Lord wanted us to invite this young man to come to America to live with us and see if it would help him in any way to get away from his own environment, which was not good as there were so many of his buddies involved in doing drugs of all kinds right there where he lived. There seemed to be an abundance of opportunities to get in trouble there at home. We mentioned this to him and told him to think about coming to live with us. Well, before we were flying out to come home, he had made up his mind. He was going to come and live with us in McDonough, Georgia, and start over with his life and try to really clean up his act. We told him that things here would be very strict for him. We would have certain rules and that he would not have much, if any, freedom to be alone. We told him that he would be inundated with the Word of God daily, but we would treat him as a member of our family. He would have freedom in our home to live with us, watch our TV, eat meals with us, go to church with us, etc., but he would not have any transportation of his own to travel about in our area. He was good with all of that at that time because he seemed to really want to make a change.

People where he lived cautioned us and begged us not to have him in our home. We were told that he would steal from us and he could get violent, but who knew what might happen to us? We were totally aware of his previous behavior and the many places he had been moved that tried to help him. In fact, my husband was part of an incident earlier on when they had placed him in a rehab center here in the Atlanta area, and Roger and another family member and friend were called to that place to try to calm him down and make him cooperate. So we were not unaware of the possibilities of his outbursts happening in our own home, but still we felt that God wanted us to try to help him.

In spite of the above, we do have some wonderful memories of this time with him and our times in the Word of God as both Roger and I mentored him daily. My time with him was always early in the morning at the kitchen table with both of us with our Bibles open, studying the Word, comparing things we found in the scriptures, and talking about many, many things that were on his heart and mind. We could see that he had a lot of experiences that had built up in his life, and probably he had never told anyone about them before. It seemed to us that these things, no doubt, led to some of his wrong choices. It was quite an interesting time for us but also very overwhelming for both of us, as one of us had to be with him at all times.

Roger would take him around with him on all of the daily routine things he had to do while I worked in our office. Roger would use that time to pour into him some life lessons and personal testimonies. He would also see that we had a nightly time of devotions before going to bed. He would bring something from the Bible, and we would discuss many prayer requests.

What was really unexpected was that after he had been here a while, he soon began to act like one of my bosses in the office! He had me writing letters for him to family and friends and various ministers he wanted to contact. I actually felt I was his secretary, too. We laughed a lot about this. He had such a great personality, you couldn't refuse him. Everyone loved this guy, and it was all of our family's prayers, hopes, and dreams that this was going to be the defining moment in his life when he was going to make it 100 percent to complete recovery from all of his addictions.

Some of the funny things I recall about having him in our home were the things he would like to eat and the hours he wanted to eat. We would go to bed at a decent time, but he would be up half the night, and at midnight, oftentimes, he would be fixing himself snacks such as sardines and crackers or ramen noodles. I guess he had learned to survive on this type of food when he was running wild and spending all of his money on drugs and booze. We laughed about the things he ate. Now, before you think that we had to buy all these sardines and ramen noodles (which are very inexpensive), or any of the food he enjoyed with us, even steaks he grilled for us, I want you to know that his parents sent money to us every single month to more than cover his expenses. They were very thankful that we were willing to try to help him, and they never ever let us spend our own funds to care for this big tall dude.

As a matter of fact, his parents expressed their gratitude to us in many different ways and were very generous toward our ministry in Albania as well. This guy was tall and skinny because he had let his health run down. He also smoked, and, of course, we didn't allow him to smoke in our house, so he would go outside in the driveway to smoke, no matter what the weather was or what time it was when he wanted a cigarette. We had an alarm system on our home, and we had told him he couldn't smoke after we went to bed and set the alarm, and he was used to that rule, but one night he completely forgot and went outside in the driveway to smoke and our alarm went off. He didn't know how to shut it off, and we were both sleeping so soundly that we didn't wake up and hear it before the police came to the house.

They saw him out in the driveway smoking and immediately asked him who he was and what he was doing there. He told them he lived there and told them whose home it was. The police didn't really believe him so they wouldn't let him go in and wake us up, but they let him stand at the far end of the hallway and holler to us and try to wake us up. Oh, it was funny for sure! We finally heard all the commotion and woke up, and Roger went out there and saw the police questioning him, asking him for his identification, etc. I stayed in the bedroom. They finally got it all straightened out and left, and then I got up, and we all had a great laugh about it. Let me tell you, it made a believer out of our friend that he could not go out and smoke after we had set the alarm at night! We had not given him the code to turn off the alarm. And we did not give it to him then either.

Soon after he came to live with us, the president of Hope for the World was taking a mission team into Brazil to do some evangelism on the streets of the cities. He had made up a team with music and some preachers. Our son, Buddy, and his best friend, Westley, were a part of that team. They were good at singing duets together, and, of course, Buddy could sing a lot of solos, too. They invited our "houseguest" to go with them so he could give his testimony of how he had a life that had been addicted to drugs and alcohol and how he had found Christ recently and wanted to serve him and was finally walking the way he knew he should as a Christian.

In fact, he had given his testimony at several churches and Jubilees where we had taken him, and he was a gifted speaker and very charismatic in his personality, and his island accent made people enjoy listening to him speak. So his parents furnished the funds for him to go on this mission endeavor, and the word came back to us when they returned that he did an awesome job of street preaching and testifying, and although there were thousands there, you could hear a pin drop when he was talking.

Well, you can see why we felt so compelled to help this young man. God truly had a hand on him and was able to use him for his glory. I can remember many services when he spoke, and mothers would come to him and talk with him about their sons who were also hooked on drugs and in trouble. Many were in prison. They found some hope by seeing and hearing our friend giving his testimony. He really seemed happy during those times.

I want to insert one paragraph before I forget it. During this time we were mentoring this young man, I can honestly say that it took much time away from our own family. I truly regret that as I look back on it. Our grandsons, Brady and Austin, were small boys then, and although they would still come over to our house and many times our friend would even play with them in special ways, like building boats, or forts outside, etc., for the most part, our attention was not on them as much as I would have liked it to be. I miss that even now as I am writing this, and I really do not know how our daughter or son truly felt about this, although they seemed to be just as hopeful that this mentoring would have eternal value. They were very kind to him and to us and felt we were ministering, but I sometimes wonder if I was doing any disservice to them by concentrating so heavily on our friend we were mentoring. I have chosen not to use his name because I want to maintain some privacy for him. We still love him and do not mean any harm to him from including his story in this book. He really has a pretty awesome story and was a big part of our lives for that period of time in 1999.

While he stayed with us, he got more and more interested in our work in Albania. Roger had gone to Albania, and the young man's mother had come to visit him at our home while Roger was gone. Well, he decided after Roger was gone a couple of days that he wanted to go on over to Albania and surprise Roger by just showing up! He knew all about the Kosovo war that was going on, and he wanted to help in any way he could with the Kosovan refugee camps, as there was a huge influx of Kosovan refugees coming into Albania because of Milosevic trying to commit genocide on that entire group of Albanians who had lived in Yugoslavia (Serbia). This was known as "the Kosovo crisis."

So the young man's mother and I began helping him make plans to go to Albania. The only way he could get there was through Italy and then by ferry over to Durress, Albania, as all the commercial planes were cancelled during that time. Roger had made his way through that same route a few days before, and there is one great tale to tell about his trip, which I will save for later! Well, we got his ticket, his mother bought his supplies and got him cash to carry on him so he would be able to minister to the refugees, and off he went. We did not warn Roger that he was coming, but our friend knew where Roger would be staying so he would be able to find him once he got into Albania.

His trip was pretty interesting and quite an adventure! He was successful in making it all the way to Durress and then getting someone to drive him to Tirana to the Stephen Center where Roger was staying. That is where he first appeared to Roger, surprising him to death! He then joined Roger, and they traveled together working with the Kosovan refugees. Roger was able to see how great he was at working in these refugee camps and helping these poor people by taking them to hospitals, feeding them meals, helping older people get from their refugee centers to doctors, etc. He wanted to stay there in Albania and continue working in that ministry, and Roger decided to let him stay.

(Side note: Our orphanage in Tirana had a wonderful professional bakery that had been donated to them by the people from Holland. Our orphans had learned how to bake bread, and they were baking over two hundred loaves of bread per day and delivering it to one of the refugee camps there in the Tirana area.)

Our friend was invaluable to the work in the Shkodra area. He did have to use interpreters part of the time, so some of our staff would have to go with him at times in order to interpret for him, but most of the time, he was on his own, making things happen in a way that made everyone truly amazed. He seemed so gifted at this type of work and a real natural. He used his own money to pay for the transport of these poor refugees to and from doctors, hospitals, etc. He bought food for many of them. He even bought food and took it to a sweet widow woman who lived next door to our missionary,

Theresa Weaver. His heart was as big as all outdoors. He had asked his folks to send him money to continually help during this time in Albania. They would send it through us, and we would wire it over to him when we sent our regular budget. He was given a small sleeping area near the main lobby at the preschool orphanage in Shkodra where he stayed. He loved all of those little orphan kids, and they truly loved him. He was tall, as I mentioned, and they would climb all over him at times like he was a jungle gym. We had many pictures coming back to us in our office of the great fun the kids had with him and he with them.

After things calmed down with the crisis, he began looking for friends apart from our staff, and unfortunately, he found himself right in the middle of some of the roughest gangs in Shkodra, Albania, really Mafia-type guys. We actually met some of them one night and could tell that they would not be the best influence on him. We were scheduled to go back again to Albania, and his parents went with us that time as they wanted to visit their son as well as see our work there in that country. They talked pretty straight to him while there and told him he had better keep his nose clean, and of course, he agreed to do so. But not too long after that, Roger got word from some of our staff that he was really going to get into trouble if he didn't pull away entirely from that group, so Roger asked him to come back to the States. He came back, and life resumed much as it had been at our home before he went.

Roger began to ease up on him a little bit when he came back from Albania and began to let him drive our old blue pickup truck. I'm not so sure that was a great idea, and we did have some incidents that led me to begin questioning some things. We soon had to take a trip by ourselves (without him), and we were gone for about a week. He had decided during that week he would go to North Carolina where we had been to a church a few weeks prior to this time. He had met a certain young woman there at that church, and we didn't know how much they had been keeping in touch since that time, but he was wanting to go there and spend a few days and get to know her better. Well, we were going to be gone, but after all, he was twenty-eight years old. We discussed this idea with his parents to see what their wishes were, because one of them could have come to our home and stayed with him if they wanted to, but there was no way we could cancel this booking to this scheduled missions conference, and it was by air to a little island in Abaco, Bahamas. We couldn't take him with us as we could not afford a plane ticket nor did the church offer to pay his way. So his parents said he could go to North Carolina, and away he went, driving our pickup truck.

When we got back home from our trip, and he returned from North Carolina, he came in telling us he was madly in love and going to marry the young woman. Wow! What a surprise! He had never been married, and we knew that he had told us that he had always hoped and dreamed of having his own family, and he did appear smitten with this young lady. We didn't know her or anything about her really, except that she had been married and had two children. We felt that he was really taking on more than he would be able to handle since he had not built up any savings, did not have a job, had not worked in years, and was still in a rehab state, so we tried to discourage this marriage based on these things alone. Well, as you can imagine, that did not set well with him, and since he had informed his parents, and they were OK with it, we had no alternative but to do all we could do to help him have a very nice church wedding. Our family took part in the music, the ceremony, the reception, everything. It was a very nice wedding celebration, and his family helped them to get all settled into an apartment not too far from us in McDonough, Georgia. We hoped that things would go well and they would have a nice Christian home as we had heard him pray for that very thing over and over again when we would have prayer time here at our home with him every night.

That was one of the other things about him that genuinely touched my heart and made me believe he had a true relationship with the Lord, his praying. He would pray for friends back home and elderly relatives who were sick, etc., and his heart was breaking as he prayed. He would actually cry when he heard that some of his old friends were suffering physically. We truly believed that he knew the Lord and that he had made some good headway toward having a wonderful life in the future, but there were many uncertainties surrounding the situation.

He did not continue in church with us, and things did not pan out really well for them. His marriage did not last very long at all, and after living through some very troublesome times, he finally moved back to his home in the Bahamas. In fact, that is where he is today, and we are thankful to say that just recently, we saw him and talked with him. He has married again and seems to still be struggling with an alcohol problem. We still love that man very much and continue to pray for him. He is working for his father, and we can only hope and pray that things will get better for him. He is now in his forties, so you can see, it has been a while since all of these things happened, and we just pray that there was something good that came from his time with us. He did tell us when we saw him recently that some of the best days of his life were spent when he was with us, but he always did know exactly what to say to make us feel good! Ha ha. He will never change in that way! We will always pray for him.

Ikim! Ikim! Let's Get Out of Here!

There is an experience that happened to Roger in his early years in Albania that could have wound up being very dangerous! When he goes to Albania, he usually manages to carry several thousand dollars on his person. These funds are to cover our own in-country expenses for hotels, food at restaurants, entertaining of staff and sometimes government directors of orphanages at meals at which time we also conduct much business surrounding the orphanages, projects to be done in the future, etc. Sometimes, he is also bringing cash to people in Albania from family members in the United States who have asked us to bring money to them as they do not have any other way to get it to them.

Well, such was the case at this particular time when he was in Albania by himself. I was not on this particular trip, so I have heard this story from him and also from some of the others who were with him on this occasion. I'll try to relate it to the best of my memory and Roger's too, as he is sitting close by as I am writing this. (Our favorite together time lately. He watches TV, and I have my laptop here on a little table in the living room right beside him, and we can chat about the things that are either on TV or in my book.)

It seems that this was one of the days he was going to spend in the northernmost city where our works are, in Shkoder. At that time, we just had one orphanage we were helping in Shkoder. It was the preschool home. The director there was Maria, and we had our American missionary, Theresa Weaver, working there in Shkoder also. Roger was taking all of our staff, including Maria and Theresa, and they were going to lunch with our staff to a very good fish restaurant about ten miles out of the city on bad, bad roads, so it seemed much further away due to the potholes in the road.

Whenever you go out to eat in Albania, and especially in those earliest days in Albania when they didn't even have electricity on a regular basis, you could spend hours just having a meal in a restaurant as they never ever prepared food ahead of time. They wait for a paying customer to come in and order, and then they pride themselves in preparing fresh food for each person. This would usually result in the meals coming out one at a time, and it taking an hour or more before everyone had their meal. You either went ahead and ate while yours was hot or, if you wanted to be really polite, you would wait and allow your meal to get cold. It was not the best situation no matter which you chose to do.

I never went back and looked at the kitchen in these restaurants, so I'm not sure just how they were cooking the food, but I'm pretty sure they were cooking on an open fire rather than trying to cook on anything as modern as an electric stove and especially since their electricity was not working so much of the time. Many times, we would go in to eat around two in the afternoon, but by the time we would leave, it would be nearly dark. This did not bother us as we got to have a lot of fellowship or conduct a lot of business during these meals. And the Albanians were used to it, so it was all "good."

Now Roger had not yet learned that in a country that is the poorest in Eastern Europe, and one that is also famous for its bandits and robbers (especially in the countryside, away from the cities), you just never, never pull out a wad of cash in a public place. Not knowing this, and having been talking with the director, Maria, about an urgent need at the orphanage, and having enough cash with him to be able to meet that need at that particular time, Roger just whipped out a wad of cash and started peeling off bills and counting hundreds of dollars to take care of that need right there and then. Well! Every Albanian at the table gasped! They started motioning him to stick that money back into his pocket quickly. It seemed they had already spotted a group of three or four men seated at the bar in that restaurant, and it was apparent that they were watching as there was an "Americano" in the group. The men appeared to be very scary to the group, and so they wanted to hurry and get out of there just as soon as possible before it would be dark as they had some distance to travel on a bad road to get back into civilization.

They settled their bill, made a dash to the old van, got in, and quickly drove away. Then they noticed that group of men also coming out and getting into their small old model Volkswagen. Immediately, when Roger's group got into the van, Maria (to whom Roger had given several hundred dollars for the needs of the orphanage) took a knife out of her purse and slit the back of the seat in the van and stuffed the money into it. She was just dead sure these men were robbers and were going to follow them and apprehend them on the road and take all of their money and possibly do them in!

"Ikim! Ikim! Driver!" which means, "let's go and hurry!" was being yelled by Theresa and Maria and all of the other Albanians in the van. We would say, "Put the pedal to the metal!" The driver took off as quickly as he could and drove just as fast as possible on those terrible potholed roads. It was really a scary time. The van was old, not in the best shape either, and they were trying to get a head start on those guys who were definitely coming along as fast as they could behind them.

They made it to Shkoder where they were dropping off Theresa and Maria and whoever else was getting out there. And they noticed that they did not see the carload of men right then, so they were glad and immediately continued on their destination to Tirana for the night, another four-hour drive away. When they arrived in Tirana, they had a phone message from Theresa letting them know that she had seen that car broken down and one of the wheels had actually come off of the axle. It was truly a God thing! He kept them from ever catching up with the van and doing anyone harm. It sort of made me think of the story of Moses being saved from Pharaoh's army when the Israelites were fleeing from Egypt! Didn't God make the wheels come off of their chariots and they dropped on their axles? Amen!

Kosovo War Memories

It was in 1999 when the Kosovo War was in progress and thousands of Kosovan refugees were migrating over the northern border of Albania into Shkodra. Many of our staff and missionary friends in Albania were working in the makeshift refugee camps assisting in feeding, clothing, medical treatment, and just generally helping as these people had fled for their lives as thousands had been killed in Kosovo under the direction of Milosevic.

At that time, they had closed the airport in Albania, and no commercial planes were allowed to go into the country. It was set apart for military flights only. Funds were not allowed to get into Albania through the usual methods, and it became necessary for Roger to personally carry the funds for our budget into Albania by hand. This alone could be very dangerous should he be overtaken by any who were either enemies of Albania or who hated Americans and our freedom, as it was not uncommon for Americans to be attacked in many countries by terrorists. To say that I was a little uneasy with him going at this time would be a great understatement. I really understood that he must go, and I also knew that I must trust the Lord for his safety, but I was truly uneasy this time because he was going to have to go in a different way than he had gone before. Instead of flying right into Tirana, Albania, he was going to fly into Rome, Italy, and then take a train to Bari (down near the boot heel of Italy); then he would take a fast ferry across the Adriatic Sea and arrive on the coast at Durress, Albania. This was a six- or seven-hour "rough" ferry ride.

I want to insert something that came to my mind when I was writing about how scared I was for Roger to make this trip this time. I opened my Bible the morning after he left home on this trip, and wouldn't you know that God had a very special scripture for me? This is what it said, right there in Proverbs 7:19-20: "For my husband is not at home. He has gone on a long journey; He has taken a bag of money with him, and will come home on the appointed day." Well, suffice it to say, I didn't worry another minute about him being on this trip.

There was a man named George, from Alabama, who worked in Washington, DC, who at the last minute heard Roger was going and had decided he wanted to go with him. Roger did not know him but had just met him at a church the week before. He had no idea what type of traveling companion he would be, but he was glad to have him come along so he would not be going entirely alone. It turned out to be quite interesting having George along. To begin with, when they had to find their way from the airport to the train station in Rome, they were pretty conspicuous as Americans. They couldn't even ask questions and get answers from people about where to find their train since neither of them spoke Italian, and it seemed that no one wanted to speak English or didn't know English. So they stuck out like a sore thumb as probably the only Americans in the crowd. However, the police helped them get on their correct train to Bari.

Then of all things, George noticed a group of three or four men that he thought were Islamic terrorists or something of the kind, and he told Roger that they kept watching them. He started referring to them as "Bin Laden's Group." He had it in his mind that they were going to attack them and rob them. He was very antsy and really making Roger a little nervous. It seemed that they followed them and even wound up boarding the same train and then even sat in the same car on the train. Oh, my goodness! This was going to be a really interesting trip, not being able to speak or understand Italian and then wondering about this group. Also, Roger had never gone this way before, and so he had no idea how long the trip would take. It was not a long distance from Rome to Bari, but he said that the train stopped every mile and picked up people and let people off. It was ridiculous! The trip took six hours. From midnight until 6:00 a.m.

Besides the strange "Bin Laden's Group," the train was also filling up with what was known as the "Freedom Fighters." They were volunteer Albanian men who had been living in European countries, or working in Italy, who were returning to Albania and would become a part of the military who would go up into Kosovo to fight Milosevic's army in this war. Well, it was quite a trip to say the least. Roger and George didn't dare try to go to sleep because of the people surrounding them and probably couldn't have slept anyway due to the many stops and starts.

They finally made it to Bari six hours later, and everyone off-boarded the train and ran to an area where there was a ticket office that would open shortly. All of the people just lined up in a horizontal line, not a line with one person behind another, but rather they were all side by side and really jammed into this space. It was crazy, Roger said. He had told George to stay outside under a tree with their luggage, as they would have to come out there anyway to board the ferry. Roger was going to stay in line to buy their ferry tickets. He stood there in this crowd where most everyone was smoking, and he was having to try to breathe—quite an effort all on its own. When they finally came and opened up the ticket counter, Roger pulled out his passport. When the bunch around him saw that he had an American passport, they immediately gave him great respect and began to push him right to the front of the line, yelling "Americano! Americano!" He couldn't believe it! He said to himself, "Wow, why didn't I flash my American passport a long time ago?" He felt like a celebrity. They were very kind to him from that point on and made sure he was at the front of every line and was even seated wherever he wanted to sit on the ferry when they boarded.

Roger had never been on one of those fast ferries known as a hydrofoil, but he had been told to take some Dramamine for motion sickness as it could be a pretty rough ride. Well, instead of just taking one Dramamine as suggested on the box, he thought that two would be better, so he took two. He told me that it seemed that everyone all over that boat was getting seasick but him. They were throwing up all over the place. His only problem was that whenever he would get up to walk to the bathroom, he was so "drunk" or "groggy" from the two pills he took, that it was a real nightmare just getting there and getting the mission accomplished and getting back to his seat. Quite a feat! He said, "You really don't want to know what it was like inside that restroom." And I didn't urge him to describe it to me. Ha! Ha!

The trip was definitely one to remember. It took six hours by ferry. The one good thing was that they never did see that particular group that George had dubbed "Ben Laden's Group" again. The Adriatic Sea was rough the whole time, and the port authority had taken everyone's passports from them when they entered the ferry, so when they arrived on shore at Durress, Albania, it took quite a while for them to call out everyone's names and return their passports. Roger and George were the last ones to get their passports returned. They were the only Americans on the ferry. They were also the last to pick up their luggage, but thankfully, as soon as they set foot in the parking area, there was Perparim, our HFTW Albanian president, and Sokrat, the driver, waiting on them. They were so glad to finally be there and be among friends and familiar faces. Since Hope for the World no longer had a guesthouse (we had sold it to a Christian Dutch group from Holland), Roger would always choose to stay at another place that was owned by a good Christian couple from Virginia. They were Chris and Laura Dakas, and they soon became our good friends. They had been among some of the very first missionaries into Albania as well and had bought a building that was in a good location on a very busy intersection in Tirana. There, they had opened up a hotel called Qendra Stefan (Stephen Center). It was a restaurant with American-style cooking and had a second floor with motel rooms. There were not too many rooms, and there were only two bathrooms which had to be shared by all of the guests. One bathroom was for the men, and one was for the women. There were two or three showers in each of the bathrooms. The Stephen Center has become one of the most popular places for American missionaries to stay when coming to Albania. Through the years, they have made many wonderful improvements to the hotel as well as the restaurant. Now, for instance, each room has its own private bathroom with a shower. All the rooms are air-conditioned. There is access to Wi-Fi, and it is much like a Starbucks where local missionaries come and hang out with their laptops and fellowship with other missionaries and visitors not only from America but from other English-speaking countries. No one is kept from coming and enjoying the Stephen Center, but the population still continues to be largely Christians gathering there. We have come to feel that it is our home while in Tirana. We love Chris and Laura as well as their Albanian manager and the workers there. We are like family with all of them.

Well, Roger had another friend from America waiting for him at the Stephen Center. That friend was Les Heath. He had already been there a few days before Roger arrived. They had planned to be there together at this time. Les also did a lot of mission work in Romania, so quite often, he would visit both countries when he came to Eastern Europe. It's really interesting when we think about where we first met Les. It was at a Bill Gaither Praise Gathering in Indianapolis, Indiana. We were there because our son, Buddy, was singing at the Praise Gathering with his group that was then traveling together as "Mullins & Company." These were the same guys Buddy had been singing with for years, ever since before Roger stopped singing with them. I remember at that particular Praise Gathering meeting Les Heath as we were walking through a long line to get something to eat. We got to talking, and he mentioned Romania. It so happened that we had been to Romania on a mission trip a little bit before that but were now working in Albania. One thing led to another, and Roger and Les connected. Les told Roger about his friend, Chris Dakas, opening a restaurant and hotel in Albania, and that's where our connection and lifelong friendship began. Les was glad to see Roger. He was a single man, divorced for many years and apparently going to stay that way, even though he had many friends trying to play matchmaker for him through the years. He liked his freedom and loved going to mission fields instead of on regular vacations. Les was a real blessing in Albania, not only to our staff but also to some of the orphans and other Albanian people he came to know. He made a huge impact on many, and we were always blessed to have him go and spend time whenever we were there, as well as other times.

Roger and Les traveled together visiting the refugee camps where the individuals and families from Kosovo were staying. They made the trip to Shkodra and spent one whole day there moving around inside a big sports center where there were thousands of refugees crammed in sitting all over the floor on mats in groups of families. The floor was totally filled with people who had escaped Kosovo, fleeing for their lives, back to their homeland of Albania. Roger and Les had Prenda, one of our staff workers, interpreting for them as they stepped gingerly between congested family groups and searched for what they hoped to be a big enough spot to place their feet. They were also helping members of our staff, as well as some of the orphans, distribute boiled eggs, bread, and water to some of the refugees. They would stop and try to speak to some of them whenever possible, but it was very noisy and hard to really carry on much of a conversation in that crowded room.

There was a young girl, who looked to be in her early teens, sitting all alone and staring blankly into space, evidently in a state of shock. Roger noticed her and wanted to see if Prenda could help him find out something about her. She was not with any adults, so she apparently didn't have any family there. It was their thinking that probably there would be many young kids who would end up moving into the orphanages as a result of this great exodus from Kosovo. They wondered if perhaps that would be the case with this young girl. They stopped and gave her some food and water and tried to speak to her. She didn't seem to want to speak, and they were about to walk away when she reached out and tugged on Prenda's shirt. She said she would like to talk with someone. What they heard from her was one of the most unbelievable stories you could ever imagine. She told Prenda the following story.

"I was sitting at the supper table with my family, my mom, my dad, my sister, and my brother. We had a baby brother in another room in a crib. Suddenly, into our house stormed some masked men from Milosovec's army. (Milosovec was the president of Yugoslavia, a very evil and ruthless man.) The masked men rushed in demanding to know what we were eating. My father answered that we were having some soup. He offered them some soup. They started wandering through the house, and they saw my baby brother. They pulled him out of his bed and cut him up into pieces with their machetes and threw his body parts on our table and said to us, 'There, now you have some meat for your soup.' They then ordered all of us out of our chairs and lined us up against the wall in the back bedroom. My father put me behind him. They began shooting, and they shot all of my family. My father's body fell down on me. The men then all ran out of the house, and I found that I was still alive and crawled out from under my father and climbed out the bedroom window and began running. The men then ran back and torched our house, and I could see it all going up in flames. I was the only one from my family saved alive, and I have been walking for many days to get here. I am here, and I am all alone with no family."

Can you imagine how this story affected Roger, Les, and Prenda when they heard it? It literally made them sick, and they felt so helpless. They offered to try to help her in any way they could, but the other Kosovans all around her would band together to help one another. In fact, in a few months, when this crisis was over and the war ended and they returned to their home country, there were absolutely no children left behind. They took all of them with them and planned to take care of them in their country. That war will never be forgotten. It was a really beautiful sight to see how the little country of Albania, which was far poorer than the country of Kosovo to which these Albanians had fled years ago, rallied to the needs of all of these Kosovan refugees and took them in, loved them, doctored them, fed them, and made sure they had their needs met. Albanians are a wonderful group of people, always ready to help those in distress, even when they have nothing much for themselves.

While I'm thinking about their helping others, I might just mention right here that during the Holocaust of the Jews by the German Nazis, Albania was a country that was a safe harbor for many Jewish refugees who came to their country. They took them in, hid them, and kept them safe. To this day, Albania is known as a great friend to the Jewish nation. Israel is one of the countries to which Albanians are free to travel with absolutely no need of a visa because of their help during that crucial time during World War II.

Meet The Zefi Family

In Prenda's Own Words

I am Prenda, and I was born on January 23, 1976, in Mesu, a village of Puke, Albania, way up in the mountains. I was the eighth child born in my family. I have five older sisters, two older brothers, and one younger brother. So as you can see, there were nine children in our family. When I was a child, we were very poor, and so, of course, we did not each have our own bedroom. Life in the village was not easy. We all had to do something to help take care of the family. I was in charge of taking the animals, cows and sheep, out to eat. I was a little shepherdess in other words. In my country, we were not allowed to mention God, but I remember that I was so interested in learning the Catholic prayers, as I had come from a Catholic family background. All of that was very hidden, and we were not allowed to tell anyone.

All of the poems I wrote at school were about Enver Hoxha, the dictator of our country. We were really taught to love him and worship him as the greatest, like God. We really thought we were so blessed to be born in Albania. When I was fourteen years old, I came to Shkodra to study foreign languages. This was in 1991, the year when communism fell and all the churches were opened again. They had been closed since 1967. I was so happy to be able to go to the cathedral here in Shkodra, the biggest Catholic church in the Balkans, and pray to the statues almost every morning before going to school.

After I finished high school, I moved from the high school dorm, which was next to the Catholic church, to the university dorm. I did not go so often to the church anymore. I did not know God's wonderful plan for me. There were some young missionaries who came to the dorm to share with us girls the plan of salvation. I did not want to listen to them. In my mind, I was a believer, and even when we were not allowed to talk about God, I was the little girl memorizing prayers.

The Bible says in Jeremiah 29:13, "And ye shall seek me, and find me, when ye shall search for me with all your heart." So on November 13, 1997, when Pastor David Hosaflook (a missionary from America) was preaching at a youth meeting, God opened my eyes, and I understood that I just believed in Jesus in my *mind*, but I had never received *him* as my Lord and Savior in my heart.

John 16:4 says, "Jesus answered, 'I am the way and the truth and the life. No one comes to the Father except through me'." This verse touched my heart. I prayed and asked God for forgiveness and asked him into my heart.

I was so happy for what happened that I could not wait to share the wonderful news with my family. However, they were really not happy with my decision, and they did not want me to go to the Baptist church. My desire and my prayers were for my family to understand the truth and to be saved. One of the reasons they were afraid of this teaching was because there was some cultish religious organization that had sprung up in our country, and people were claiming to follow the Bible but were committing suicide. My parents were afraid I may be getting into something like that.

After I graduated, God blessed me by allowing me to become a part of Hope for the World. I started working at the baby orphanage in the year 2000. How excited I was. The same year God had another *big* blessing for me. Fredi (my future husband) came to work with Hope for the World at the school-age orphanage. I thought he was a very handsome guy, but it took us a little time to get to know one another. We really spent the most time together when we were both taking the driver's training course. We planned that so we would get to spend time together, as in my country there was not such a thing as "dating" in public or so that anyone knew you were actually dating, not until later, when things were really getting serious. But we fell in love, and we got married November 29, 2000. Now we have three wonderful children. Of course, life is full of blessings and challenges, but I would not change anything.

My mother passed away on Christmas Day the same year I married Fredi. That was a very, very difficult time for me. Cherie came to Albania for a visit the next spring, and she and I went to spend the night on Easter at my sister's house where the other sisters were all gathered. It was a special day of mourning, as it was the first Easter without our mother. God used it in a great way. Cherie was sharing the gospel with them the whole time, and Mrike and Dila received Christ in their heart that evening and Bardhja the next morning. What a blessing!

Some thoughts from Cherie:

Prenda came to visit us in our home in America, soon after she had met Fredi Zefi. He was a new employee of ours and very handsome. I had not met him yet, but we trusted our staff worker, Theresa Weaver, with the hiring of Fredi as she knew him well and knew that he was a young Christian and wanted to really do something with his life. He had been teaching French in schools in Albania. He already had his college education and was well equipped to be a good role model for the children in the school-age orphanage of Albania. I had noticed that emails I would receive from Prenda would mention Fredi quite often, ha ha. So I began to realize that there may just be a "love connection" taking place there. Well, she came with Theresa to America and spent her first days here with us. We were getting ready to go to Albania, so Prenda asked me to "check him out" when I got there to see what I thought about him as a good prospect for her future.

Now, our first place to go whenever we go to Albania is Shkodra, the northernmost point of all of our works in Albania. So we went to Shkodra, and one of the places we took our group to see and to have a meal was at the Rosafa Castle, way up high overlooking the city of Shkodra. The weather had been rainy, and we cannot drive up and park on the property. We have to always park at the foot of a long hill, and we must walk up on cobblestones to the castle. It is quite a trek for old people, to tell you the truth. And even more of a trek when it is wet and the stones are slippery, and if you have bad knees.

So all of that being said, when we arrived there (with Fredi along with us as a sort of "tour guide" for our group, as he spoke English very well), we got out of the van and started walking up the hill. Fredi grabbed hold of me, took my arm in his, and held me so strong and safely that I hardly noticed I was climbing a hill. This was my very first time to meet this young man. I was thinking in my head the whole time, *If Prenda doesn't catch this young man, she's absolutely crazy*. He was the epitome of gentleness, kindness, respectfulness, and helpfulness. My goodness, I had never met any young man that could even begin to measure up to him in all of the wonderful attributes he displayed. Now, could it be he was really trying hard to impress me? I have no idea, since he knew Prenda had just been with me and probably surmised that she and I had talked about him some. But no, now that I have known him all these years and watched his life with the children in the orphanages, and now as a father of three beautiful children, I realize that was just who he was. We are so blessed to have Prenda and Fredi as a part of our organization. We pray that they will be with HFTW all of their lives and serving the Lord with us in Albania, reaching orphans and many others on a daily basis.

Prenda has been like another daughter to me. She began with us as a young girl and is now a wonderful mother of three children of her own, plus a foster child from the orphanage. She has been the very best worker we could have ever asked for in the baby orphanage and day care center in Shkodra. All of the workers love her, although it was not that way at the very beginning. They came to love her as they saw that her heart and her life were such an example of God's love to the children and to them as well.

We truly have another whole family in Albania. We love not only Fredi and Prenda but also their children, Edona, Tedj, Reuel, and Klodjan. God has gifted them with much talent in so many areas of their lives. We can see that these youngsters already have the heart of young missionaries. They care for others, their friends in school, the orphans, everyone. We thank God for the wonderful lives they will have ahead of them because they have been brought up in this Christian home of Fredi and Prenda Zefi. Praise the Lord that the Gospel is now allowed in Albania. It is no longer under the communist regime and atheism. This family is doing their part to bring many to Christ, and it began with their own family members.

Fredi's Testimony

I am Prenda's husband, Alfred Zefi. I was raised in the Catholic tradition of my family in Tropoja. In our family, while growing up, we did not practice religion as it was prohibited by the dictatorship of the time under the dictator, Enver Hoxha. Albania was known as the only atheist country in the world. In 1967, all the churches and mosques were closed, and they turned the buildings into sports centers or government offices. The only person that was worshiped by Albanians was the dictator.

In 1991, communism fell. Albania started to practice religion again. In 1992, I moved to Shkoder to study foreign languages as, in my hometown, we did not have a high school for learning languages. I lived in a dorm (a place to live while studying when you came from other towns) for four years. The first year, I was invited by some Christians to the cinema to watch the *Jesus* movie. I went to see it. At the end, they distributed New Testaments for all the people who were invited. I really liked the movie, and it made me think for a while, but after that day, I totally forgot and did not think any more about it. In the dorm, we had four students in one room. Arben, one of my roommates, started being distanced from us. Every day, he would read a book and listen to some songs. The book he was reading was the Bible. I made fun of him and teased him a lot, asking him, "Are you going to be a Catholic priest?"

Arben shared with me the Gospel. He told me that he had believed in Jesus and invited me to the church meetings. I was living a bad life and enjoying it. After many invitations, I decided to go to a church meeting. The striking thing for me was the warmth that I felt in the presence of that group of people. I even met the missionary, David Hosaflook, after the church meeting. We had a good talk with him and Arben. I was very skeptical about what they told me. I had many questions about God. Instead of giving me their opinions in answering my questions, they would open the Bible and give me answers. It took me many meetings and discussions before understanding about this "new religion." In 1994, one night in my room, while reading and thinking, I gave my life to Jesus, and I invited him to be my personal Savior and Lord. I did not have a choice. I couldn't escape from making that decision that night. Since then, my life has never been the same. I started being faithful to church meetings and started growing in knowledge and obedience to him.

After I was saved, my first mission field was under my own roof, my family. I went back to my house and shared the Gospel with my older brother, Astrit. He had many questions, and I did not have answers for many of his questions, so I invited Pastor David to come to my home and share the Gospel with Astrit and my whole family. There are eight kids in our family, six brothers and two sisters. David came to our home, and after many visits, my older brother Astrit was saved, and now he pastors the Bible Baptist Church in Tropoja, Albania. It was during the five years after I was saved that God used his servants, David, Beni, Jeff Bartell, Theresa Weaver, and many other new Albanian believers, to share the good news with my family. The last person in my family who gave his life to the Lord was my father. I am very thankful to the Lord for being gracious and saving all my family including my brothers and sisters, father, and mother very soon after my salvation.

In April of 2000, I was teaching French in the high school of Fierze-Tropoje, when Theresa Weaver, who was a missionary with Hope for the World, came to me and asked if I would be interested in working with HFTW in Shkoder at the school-age orphanage. Of course, I had to finish the school year, which ended in June, but I went to Shkoder to visit the orphanage and just to see closely about this opportunity.

THE MAKING OF A WONDERFUL LIFE

When I walked into the school-age orphanage, I met the kids and some of the staff. There were eighty-four abandoned kids during that time who lived in that particular institution. Around thirty-five workers were working there. I saw that this place was a great mission field. I decided to be a part of the HFTW staff, and since then, I have dedicated my life to this great ministry. In the same year of 2000, I met my wife, Prenda. She was also working for HFTW at the baby orphanage. On November 29, 2000, we got married, and God has blessed us with three kids, a daughter, Edona, and two sons, Tedi and Reuel. We are also new foster parents of one of the orphan boys from the baby orphanage. His name is Klodjan. So we are a family of six at the present time.

In the first four years, I worked as a sponsorship coordinator for the school-age orphanage. Since that time, I have been HFTW director for the Shkodra branch working with the baby orphanage, preschool orphanage, school-age orphanage, and center of development. For me, being able to bring joy to the hurting kids is such a tremendous ministry and blessing. Celebrating their birthday, taking them to different places and doing different activities, improving the quality of their lives with better food, better clothes, better sleeping, and living conditions, providing school supplies, and helping them to follow different courses like painting, music, and sports are so much fun. However, the most important part is sharing with them the message that brings *hope*. We share it not just to them but also to the staff and to our region as well. God has allowed us through the years to see many of the kids come to know Jesus as their personal Savior through weekly Bible classes. Ministering to the orphans and widows is a call from God's Word. Discipling the ones that get saved has been and still is an important part of our ministry.

Throughout the years, we have been through many challenges and hard times, but God's presence has been with us. He will never leave us nor forsake us but will always lead us through our challenges for his honor and glory. Ministering through HFTW alongside servant leaders like Roger and Cherie, Buddy and Kerri Mullins, and Cindy Howard is a great privilege and a pleasant walk. Thinking about his works in the past, we look forward to what he will do in us and through us for his glory in the days ahead.

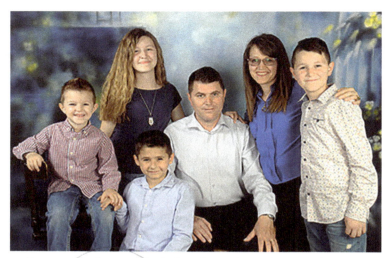

Front—Klodjan—A little boy from the orphanage that they are able to foster as their child. He grew up in the baby orphanage where Prenda works Family—Reuel, Edona, Fredi, Prenda, Tedi.

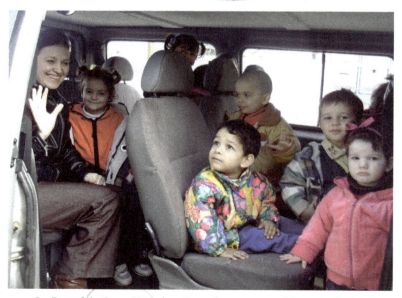

In Prenda's Own Words—Prenda is pictured here with the children from the Children's Orphanage where she works in Shkoder. This was a very special day called "Children's Day".

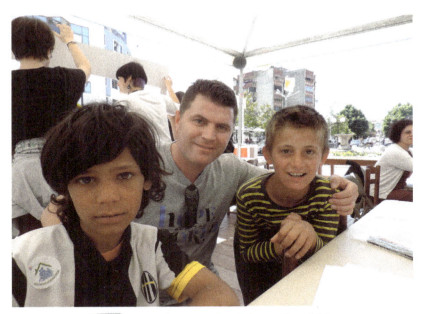

Fredi here with a couple of the orphan kids.
All the kids love Fredi and he loves them.

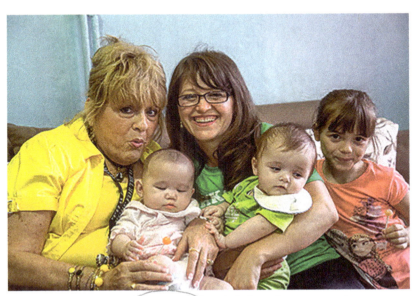

Prenda and me with babies from
The Shkoder Baby Orphanage

From Mirela's Heart

My name is Mirela Ymeraj, and I was born in Shkoder, Albania on May 20, 1977. As you have heard, our country was under communism, and it was very difficult because people were afraid to talk, for fear they would be reported to the government. We were not allowed to have the choice of believing in God or being a Christian or a Muslim. We had to stand in line to shop, and there was very little food in every shop. You sometimes had to stay hours in line, and then many times, you would not get anything. In our very small apartment lived my grandparents, my parents, me, and my three sisters, eight of us in all. My mother and father both worked, but it was very difficult to make a living. My father worked as a construction worker, building houses and apartment houses for the Albanian government, and since it was under communism, he got paid very little. Had he been able to be paid the wages people earned in the other countries, we would have been a rich family. My mother was a schoolteacher, and she was paid very, very little. Under communism, everyone was on the same level. Everyone made the same amount of money, and everyone was extremely poor. Our earnings were about the equivalent of twenty-five dollars per month.

My grandmother grew up as a Catholic, and she believed in Jesus. She would teach me about Jesus, but my mom would hear her and would not allow her to do this because my mom was an atheist by that time, under the communistic teaching. Our whole country had turned atheist. The communist wall fell when I was about fourteen or fifteen years of age. It was at this age that I saw a Bible for the first time in my life, let alone held one in my hand or read it. I had seen it in the Baptist church, and that is where I first heard the Gospel. I was very blessed, as there was an Albanian couple who would invite me to go with them to the Bible Baptist Church in Shkoder. I first refused to go as I was going to the Catholic church like my grandmother's teaching. But this couple kept inviting me to go with them for more than one year, so after that long time of their asking me, I decided to go.

It was a day they were having baptism at the church, and there I met missionary David Hosaflook, who was the pastor of the Bible Baptist Church, and he and all of the church welcomed me and were very friendly. I really enjoyed all the praying and the friendship I felt there that day. I remember that I was invited to go again, and my mom would be very upset with me because our prayer meeting was late, and it would be dark when I came home. Pastor David had to return to the United States, so we had a missionary couple who came especially for us. They were very wonderful people, Pastor Neal and Don Alice Smith. They were so very sweet and spent time with me as my grandma did. They would pray for me and with me. They needed someone to translate for them, and as I knew English, I was able to help, and I would be in all of the services that we had on Sunday, Wednesday, and Friday.

I remember it was at prayer meeting one Wednesday night, and after the message, Pastor Neal asked us to close our eyes, and he asked if there was anyone who wanted to accept the Lord Jesus as their personal Savior, and my heart started beating really fast, and I raised my hand. He was crying, and I was crying too, from happiness. He hugged me and prayed for me and with me, and that was the wonderful time of my accepting Christ as my Savior. *He is my strength, and I have no fear because of him in my life!*

Soon after that, I met Theresa Weaver, a missionary with Hope for the World to the orphans in Shkoder. I met her there at the Bible Baptist Church. She was the first missionary I came to know personally, and I am so thankful to her for the way she spent a lot of time with me teaching me many scriptures. She was an awesome mentor to me and teacher to the orphans. She and I became like sisters, and we truly were and still are sisters in Christ. She was a great blessing to me for many years, and it was through her that I got my job working for Hope for the World. My parents had no jobs at that time, and I had been working as a waitress in a restaurant when Theresa was looking for someone to hire to work with her in the orphanages. I was eighteen years of age at that time, almost nineteen.

In the beginning, my job was working right beside Theresa, translating for her, spending time with the orphans, etc. Our main focus was to teach the kids about Jesus. We read a lot of books and taught Christian songs to them, and I love to sing, so that was really something I enjoyed. I had never met the directors of Hope for the World from America at that time. It was in the year 1996 when I first met Roger and Cherie Mullins. Although it was my first time to meet them, I felt like we had known each other all our lives. They were so kind and loving to me, and when I told my family about them, they loved them too. I remember that I had prepared a nice program especially for them with the kids of the orphanage. It is still a very sweet and exciting thing for me to remember.

In January of 1997, there began a very scary time in Albania, as we had a civil disorder known as the Albanian Rebellion which broke out in our country. This caused civilians to take to the streets in protest of the government which had allowed a "Pyramid Scheme" to take place, resulting in the people losing millions of dollars. It was a huge civil unrest, and I remember as I would ride my bicycle to work at the orphanage, I would hear bullets being fired from guns all around. I was afraid for my own personal safety at times. There was not much food to buy at that time, and again, you had to stand in line for a couple of hours just to buy bread and other things to eat. The orphans were afraid, and we tried to do things with them to help calm them and to keep them from freaking out and being scared. Men would stand watch in the neighborhoods at night, taking turns. This uprising lasted for a little over six months.

It was about this time, when I was twenty years old, one of my neighbors had been planning to kidnap me. I did not know this at that time. But this was happening to girls in Albania, and they were being sold into bondage and sent to Italy. My neighbor's family and my family were friends and had a very good relationship. His mom would spend a lot of time in my home. I learned that he had told some other guy to tease me and flirt with me while I would be going to work every day, so that I would ask him (my neighbor) to help me with this guy.

It was the next day, as I was going to work, he came to me in a car beside the road and said, "Come on, get in my car, so this guy will see you with me and then I will tell him not to disturb you anymore." So trusting him as my neighbor, I got into his car, and he locked me in with him and took me to some house, I did not know, where he and others kept me for some days. (I do not like to remember this, as he was planning to sell me and send me to Italy.) After some days in the Shkoder apartment, they drove me to the city of Vlore, which is a few hours away, and on the coast of the Adriatic Sea. I was very afraid and very uncooperative and praying all the time for God to keep me safe. One of the guys I met there was another guy from my neighborhood, named Herton. He was a *big guy*! He was feeling very sorry for me, and he wanted to help me escape and get back home. He told me to not be afraid; he would help me get home. I have totally blocked out some memories of this incident, but I do know that Herton stood by his word, and he made them take me back to Shkodra. He was not afraid to confront anyone, and because of his size, no one would mess with him. Herton came from a very different background than me. He actually had to fight with the other guy in order to get this accomplished, but he did that. He fought to protect me and to get me back home. He made them bring me close to my home, and I got out of that car and ran for my life to get home again. I have not shared this story with many people, and at that time, I was in such a state of shock I could not even speak of it. I know that all of the people connected with Hope for the World were praying for me. They had no idea what had happened to me, where I was, and why I didn't come back to work at the orphanage. I really was unable to return for a while until I had recovered from this incident. Even then, I did not tell them what had happened to me. Not until recent years have I been able to share this, but I am thankful to God and to Herton that I am safe.

Herton came to my parents a couple of years after this incident and asked them to let me marry him. We married when I was twenty-three years old. I have two sons now. Hermes who was born in November of 2000 and Naimir who was born in 2005. Hermes was my first joy and the one who made me a mom. He is a very sensitive boy, intelligent, and kind. Naimir is also a very good boy and smart as well. I am so proud that both of them love to go to church with me, and it is my prayer that they will always live their lives for Jesus.

I have continued to work for Hope for the World all of these years, since I was a teenager. I am a sponsorship coordinator for them. I love working with the children of the orphanages. I know it is a job that God had for me and was in his plan for my life. Every single day, I try to show them God's love and also be a testimony to government personnel who work in the orphanage. I pray for them, and many of them have attended my church at times. I am still a member of the Bible Baptist Church, and I enjoy being a part of the worship music program there. I also am involved in the women's meetings and other church meetings.

Times have been very difficult for me as my husband does not work and provide for the family, and so it all depends on me. There have been times when he has been in jail, and that was a huge burden for me as well. But I thank God that *God is my strength*; I am strong because *he is strong*. He *is my everything*! Life is not all about material blessings of food, clothing, and fancy stuff, but it is all about *him*. With Jesus, all things are possible. I am thankful to him for all of his blessings that have come to me. Of course, I sometimes get upset that as a mother I may not be able to furnish everything for my boys that they would like to have, but I have learned so much working in these orphanages. I have so much to be thankful for. My smile comes from God. *He is my joy and my peace.*

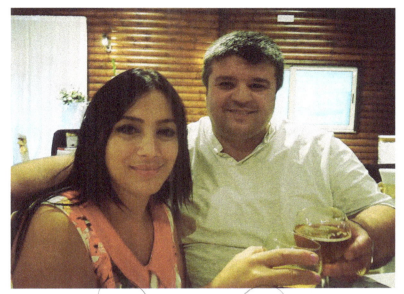

Mirela and her husband, Herton

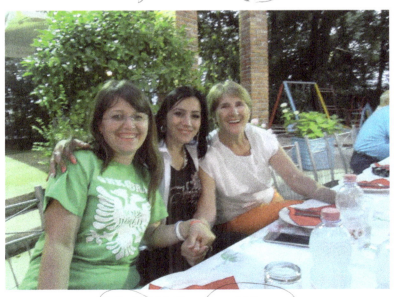

Mirela with Prenda and Nirvana
Nirvana is the wife of our employee, Nikolin.

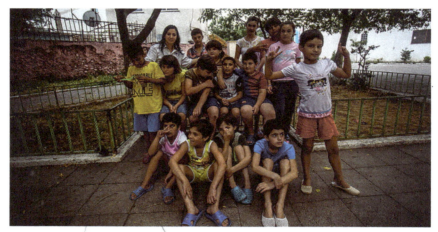

Mirela with some of her kids from the orphanage in Shkoder.
She taught them Bible and wonderful Christian songs.

Caught in a Blood Revenge

Editor's note: I wanted to follow up Mirela's story with a very interesting, yet painful, story about her husband, Herton. You noticed in her story that it appears that she is the only breadwinner for the family. Her income from Hope for the World is what takes care of her and her husband and two sons, and that is true. What she did not share with you, but has given me the opportunity to write here, is about the main reason that her husband has not been gainfully employed and working to care for his family. I ask you to pray for them in this regard.

After Herton had rescued Mirela and gotten her returned safely to her family, he began to come and talk with her. He came to know her family and spent a great deal of time there with them. He was, of course, preparing to ask them to let him marry Mirela. One time, while he was there, a knock came on the door of their home. A man was there asking for Herton and telling him that his father had been shot and was at the hospital. Herton immediately left and went to see what had happened. He went to the hospital, and his father was undergoing some surgery at that time, but he did not survive. He died there in just a few minutes from bullet wounds. This began a blood feud, also known as blood revenge, between Herton's family and the family of the man who killed his father. Blood feuds are still practiced to a great extent in northern Albania. You see, there is a set of traditional Albanian laws that date back to the fifteenth century. It is a system of justice that focuses on honor, guilt, and vengeance. It is written in a book known as the Kanun. "Spilled blood must be met with spilled blood." This is what is found in the Kanun. It threatens thousands of families in upper Albania and, in particular, in the Shkoder area where Herton and Mirela were living.

It is literally the practice of "an eye for an eye and a tooth for a tooth." The police have done very little to prosecute or imprison the people who commit these types of killings. Sometimes, they are only in prison for a few months, if at all. I have read recently that there are as many as two thousand families affected by this type of feud presently and over eight hundred children are not in school due to this practice.

What happens when there is a murder of someone in a family, under the Kanun's teachings? It is then all right for a member of that family to go and kill the murderer or even other members of the family of the killer. Even young children are not exempt from the danger of being killed. What happens is that it makes families (especially men and boys) become prisoners behind the walls of their own homes. The reason these feuds are mainly between men is because under the Kanun, women are referred to derogatorily, and their lives are thought to have not a lot of value other than bearing children. Victims of a blood feud do not dare to go out even on their own streets, much less go out in society or go to work in the public. They are always afraid for their lives. They are constantly hiding. This is what took place for Herton. He, of course, wanted to avenge his father's death and carry on the custom of his country, but he did not. But he went into hiding because if the killer's family saw him out, they would be on the defense thinking he would kill them and so they might kill him. He did, however, go ahead and marry Mirela, but that feud then entered into their marriage which has been very difficult.

The Albanian government has downplayed this problem, and the police claim that cases of blood revenge are falling dramatically with only a couple of hundred or so reported in the region since the fall of communism in 1991. The government has put stronger penalties for blood feud crimes, and perpetrators face a maximum prison sentence of, sometimes, up to forty years.

Herton came to a service once when we were in Albania, and our pastor, Ralph Easterwood, was preaching in New Hope Baptist Church in Tirana. He preached a powerful sermon on salvation, and at the time of the invitation, Herton told Mirela, "I don't want this in my life anymore" (referring to the fear he lived with, in the blood revenge feud). "I'm going to raise my hand to be saved." He raised his hand for prayer.

I had not seen Pastor Ralph give this type of invitation before, but he went further with the invitation. He said, "If you truly meant it when you raised your hand, I want you to look at me right now. Look into my eyes." He told us later, Herton looked right up at him, straight into his eyes. Pastor Ralph went a step further. He said, "If you are tired of your life of sin and you really want to give it all to Jesus and be saved today, stand to your feet."

Herton was the only person who stood to his feet that morning. Pastor Ralph then told him to come down front, and Herton very humbly and obediently came to the front of the church. He is a huge guy! We were all crying, as we knew Herton really needed to come to know Christ as his Savior. We had all been not only praying for him but, witnessing to him, many times one-on-one. So what a blessed time it was for all of us that day. Mirela was also crying tears of joy, and we were all really looking forward in great anticipation to what God would do in his life. He did make a profession of faith on that Sunday morning.

For a while, Herton went to church with Mirela, and he was discipled by missionary pastor, David Hosaflook, who took a great interest in helping him grow spiritually. He even encouraged him and helped him find some types of work to do. Brother David also taught him from the scriptures in Romans 12 where it says, "Beloved do not avenge yourselves, but rather give place to wrath; for it is written, 'Vengeance is Mine, I will repay', says the Lord." Also, our HFTW Albanian president, Perparim, counseled with Herton and tried to help him during this time. After this godly counsel, Herton took them to his uncle's house where they talked and went from there to the home of the man who had shot Herton's father. There, they met with a group of fifteen to twenty men for the purpose of resolving this blood feud between the families. An elderly man, acting as chief of the reconciliation, conducted this meeting. Herton did this on his own, really without the blessing of his mother or sisters, as they were still very angry.

Herton has not really found any job that he will commit to though he has tried a few. He did go out and seek gainful employment once in the last couple of years that I know of, but that job resulted in a bad experience for him which landed him in jail for a while which made life 'en more difficult for Mirela, as she had to bring him food regularly to the jail as well as work and take care of their boys.

We still love Herton, and we pray for him and send word to him through Mirela that we love him and that God still loves him and that he needs to get back into fellowship with God and with fellow Christians in his town. He just needs to go to 1 John 1:9 and ask for cleansing, and God will do that. All of us sin and need cleansing on a regular basis. He does send word that he reads his Bible, which is good news to us, but I am asking you, my readers, to please pray for him. He's a sweet man. I love him so much, and he's like a giant teddy bear when you look at him. He is actually the biggest Albanian man I have ever met, and I'd love to see him have a happy and full life in Christ and lead his family in that way too.

I have read that concerning these blood feuds in Albania, there is a Committee of Nationwide Reconciliation, but even when people call them and go through some form of reconciliation, it seems that people have gotten away from the Kunan and don't obey the rules anymore. They just seem to make up their own. There isn't even any respect for the age of the children involved. And although homes were once a safe haven or shelter, that is no longer the truth. But we can say the same thing about our country in these times in which we live. The Bible tells us that things will get worse the closer we get to the end of the age. In II Chronicles 7:14, it tells us that "If My people who are called by my name will humble themselves and pray and seek My face, and turn from their wicked ways, then I will hear from heaven and will forgive their sin and heal their land." This is what the whole world needs! But it begins with each individual!

Albanian Adoptions

In the years we have been in Albania, we have seen many adoptions of Albanian orphans. We are very pleased to say that many of them have been adopted into wonderful Christian families in America. Of course, they are also adopted by great families from some of the European countries. In most recent years, we have been blessed to see Albanian families adopting children from the orphanages. However, many children have been adopted from the homes that we have been ministering to since we began in 1994. Hope for the World has never been an adoption agency, but because of our ministry in Albania, many Americans have visited the country on mission trips to participate in various ministries, building and restoration projects, etc. Many have also made the tour of orphanages with us through the years, just to see all the work we have been doing in Albania and to get a heart for the ministry. It has been through these initial visits to Albania that many friends have been prompted to adopt an Albanian orphan. There have also been some American missionaries we know who have adopted children from the orphanages of Albania. It has truly been a thrill to see the way God has provided for these children who would otherwise have had no hope for a future or opportunity to further their education, etc. Some of the children adopted have had physical needs, and the adoptive parents have brought them to America and taken care of these needs. Some of the adopted children have kept in touch with us through the years they have been in America. It is always a thrill for us to get a letter or Facebook message from one of them telling us some of the wonderful things going on in their lives. I wanted to put some of these good stories into my book, and at this point, I do not know how many I will receive, but I will begin with one I just received the other day from a young lady. She was Rozana and was in the orphanage in Shkodra, Albania, when she was a little girl, during our early years working in Albania. She keeps in touch with us regularly, and I am happy to include what I just received from her recently. Here it is:

Rozana's Story

I remember living in the orphanage in Shkodra and wondering if I would ever have a home and a family. My best friend since as early as I can remember got adopted. She was five, and I was seven at the time. I remember it so clearly. I was so happy for her, but I was scared for me. At that time, I had transitioned to the big kids orphanage. It was even scarier without my best friend. I did have two brothers, and I was in the middle, and we all grew up in the same orphanage, so at least I had them with me, I thought.

I first came to know Jesus through Fredi and Prenda who worked for Hope for the World. They took us to church on Sundays and kept us out of trouble. They were so kind, giving, and full of love and hope. They even brought us to their home on occasions, and we could spend the night there. They would play games with us and make us a nice meal. It was such a treat! Then when I got my first Bible, I began reading it before bed each night and praying for a family, for a home. I remember seeing America on the news and thinking, *I'll never be able to go there*. Then I heard there was a family that was interested in adopting me. I was beyond happy! God was real, I thought, He is answering my prayer!

Then two years went by and I hadn't heard anything, and I began to lose hope. I remember asking Prenda, and she said that my dad wouldn't let me go. She thought that I, at age eleven, should convince him that this is what will be best for me and there is no future and no opportunities if I stayed in the orphanage, and that if he'd let me go, I could help them financially. So I talked to my father. It was a sad conversation, and I had to beg him to let me go. I knew it was hard for him. I knew he loved me. He visited me every month, and he gave us whatever money he could give so we could treat ourselves to candy. He just could not financially support us. I praise him for doing the hardest thing a father could do, let his daughter go to the unknown, but hope for the best for her. I could not have asked for a better adoptive family. I have truly been blessed. My parents have shown nothing but love and patience toward me. They had two other children of their own, both younger than I, and still they were able to love this young, almost twelve-year-old girl who came from Albania with an unknown past. My adoptive parents had courage and faith. I know it wasn't easy for them, but they kept believing in me and loving me unconditionally, and they kept reminding me that they loved me just the same as their biological kids. I wasn't the perfect child, but to me, they were the perfect parents. I thank God every day for them. My whole family has been nothing but a blessing. I still talk to my brothers in Albania through Facebook. I help them as much as I can financially. I send money to Brother Roger and Cherie at the Hope for the World Albania office, and they get it over to them. I know that God has the perfect plan for us all, and I believe one day we will be together again. They are always in my mind and prayers.

So here I am, living in sunny Southern California, in this cute little beach town called Dana Point. I am a hairstylist in Laguna Beach, California. I owe my life to God. I don't know what or where I would be if I hadn't received Jesus Christ as my Savior when I was in the orphanage in Shkodra. I would not be here right now. I am so very thankful to Hope for the World. God is working wonders through them.

I appreciate Rozana sharing her testimony with me. Since she wrote this and sent it to me, we have had family members who had seen her story in our newsletter. They had personal friends living right there in the same city in California where Rozana is living. As a matter of fact, the old gentleman and his wife who live there wanted to make an acquaintance with her, as the gentleman had been raised as an orphan here in America. He thought it would be interesting to compare their stories. This has happened, and I was so happy to learn that it was a very sweet experience for Rozana as well as for this lovely couple. It is so interesting the way God puts people in our lives in one country, and then they wind up over here in America connected with others with similar backgrounds as theirs. We appreciate Rozana so much and the way she loves her father and brothers and is so faithful to send money over to help them on a regular basis. What a blessing she is! Little did they know, when they allowed her to be separated from them, and adopted by an American family, one day they would look to her for their needs, and God would allow her to help in this amazing way! If there is one lesson we have learned during the years of working with Albanian people, it is that they truly love and care for their own families.

There are many, many children who have been adopted through the years, and although I would love to be able to put all of their stories in my book, time and space will not permit. If we could sit down together and chat, we could talk on this subject all day long and never get through.

Miracle of "Night of Hope"

We have written throughout this book how we were searching for just the right place in Albania to be able to have a very special place to help the teenaged orphans complete high school and prepare them for their adult life in Albania. You remember that we met with the prime minister's wife one time and tried to get her to have the government just "give us" some property that is empty and not being used in Albania. There are many properties of this type in their country. These properties had been confiscated from individual family and business owners under the communist government and had been used by the leaders during the years they were under this regime. There are very beautiful pieces of property and huge buildings with housing, restaurants, and meeting rooms. They were truly gorgeous places and were only accessible to the *elite* of the communist era.

There were also other pieces of property that were already owned by other NGOs from European countries. We had found one of them and learned that it was for sale. In fact, Roger took a group of his friends who were businessmen in Georgia who were making up an advisory board for us at that particular time and for the express purpose of helping us to make good decisions regarding purchasing property in Albania. Since Roger had never been a businessman, he felt the need to call upon a wonderful group of friends who were both Christian and were experts when it came to buildings, construction, land values, etc. They would meet on a regular basis, and Roger would share with them what we were trying to do in Albania. If there was an opportunity to buy something that would work for the teen center, we had hoped to open he would share that with these men to get their expert opinion.

There was one property in particular that I remember going to see along with Roger and some of our businessmen friends. It really looked like it could be very promising for us. It was being used in an agricultural way most of the year, raising some livestock but also raising beautiful flowers, etc. Then, in the summer months, it was being used by Christian groups in Albania as youth camps. The property was owned by someone from England, and we met with him and discussed the possibility of Hope for the World purchasing the property. It really seemed very promising to us at the start, but then as we began to get serious about making an offer, the price suddenly doubled, and that let us know it was not God's will for us. So once more, we found ourselves "still looking" and "still praying."

Along with praying and looking, we knew we had to do some type of large fund-raiser in America to purchase any land that we found in Albania. A man in our church who was on our advisory board and who had been to Albania with us more than once began to talk with us about the possibility of having a large banquet in Atlanta. We would invite hundreds of people to attend and see just how much money we could raise in order to buy property. Tony Middlebrooks and his wife, Edie, were gifted at organizing fund-raiser banquets for nonprofit organizations. They had done so before, and they were ready to do one for Hope for the World Albania. It wasn't long before heads came together and plans began to be drawn up to have an event at the Georgia Aquarium in Atlanta in their large banquet room which would seat nine hundred people for a lavish sit-down meal.

I cannot say enough about the way God allowed it to come together under Tony and Edie's direction along with tons of help from our wonderful friends and fellow church members at Glen Haven Baptist Church. The plans began to grow and develop, and Roger and I were amazed at what was coming together. We had never been a part of the corporate world and had never seen anything on this scale before. We were praying and doing a lot of the detail work here in the office, and helping in all the ways we could, but it was really all new ground for us. In dealing with the Georgia Aquarium, we found out that in order to have an event to fill up the room with nine hundred people for a banquet, we had to use their caterer, none other than the renowned Wolfgang Puck, the finest. We also learned that we had to put up a "good faith" deposit of $100,000 in advance. Oh, my goodness! I could not believe that and felt that would be the end of our planning. But no! That did not stop our fearless leaders! They had us begin right away getting the tickets printed and selling tickets to individuals, corporations, churches, and businesses. They were reaching out to everyone in many different directions to get this money together for the deposit. It was amazing to see how God provided quickly, and we were able to get that deposit in hand. Yes, we got it to them by the required deadline for the deposit. We were on our way to an awesome "Night of Hope" at the Georgia Aquarium to be held on November 2, 2006.

I really do not have the words to tell you what a wonderful help our pastor at that time, Ralph Easterwood, was in supporting this event. He wrote a beautiful letter inviting every one of our church members to attend this Night of Hope. He also mentioned it many times in the church services leading up to this time. Also, many of our friends at church who have their own businesses were a huge part of providing the funds by buying full tables for the evening and then filling them with friends and family members. We were blessed to have Mr. Truett Cathy, the founder of Chick-fil-A, as our guest speaker for the evening. He never goes anywhere without bringing gifts with him. There were little black and white cows at every plate and many, many gift cards for free Chick-fil-A sandwiches. His speech that night was so very inspiring as he has built his own business on godly principles and has been a great testimony in the corporate world of America for many years. We were so blessed to have him speak that evening. Also in attendance as a part of the evening was our Hope for the World president, Jimmy Franks, and his wife, Janice. We were so happy to have them there to represent Hope for the World which began ministering in the early 1990s in Albania. Another wonderful special guest was one of our own Albanian staff members, Nikolin Lekaj, from Shkodra, Albania. He and his wife had come to visit in our home and were there just at the right time for this event.

On the program that evening, we were happy to have DJ Michael Stuart from Radio Station J93.3 as our emcee for the evening. Wes Sarginson of 11Alive News was there to conduct our live auction. Music for the evening was provided by the powerful vocals of "Everyday Driven," a group made up of our son, Buddy Mullins, and his wife, Kerri, Channing Eleton at the keyboard and long-time friend, Paul Lancaster. We were also blessed by a very special couple, John Herring and his wife, Jennifer, who had been faithful business partners in our vision for the future of the orphans of Albania. John and Jennifer had not only visited Albania with us, but they wound up adopting a precious little girl from one of the orphanages there. What awesome friends they have been to Hope for the World.

This event proved to be a wonderful blessing in clearing the sum of $200,000 for Hope for the Future to be able to purchase property in Albania to begin our Hope Center for Teens one day. At the time of this event, we thought we were very close to purchasing the property in Albania; however, as we have learned through the years in working for the Lord, *our* timing is not always God's timing. We put those funds aside and continued on our search for just the right place and continued to pray for God to open the right doors for us in Albania.

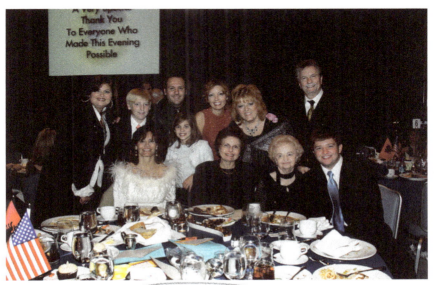

Night of Hope—Family Group…
Such a special Night at the GA Aquarium
These are all family members…
Roger and I were blessed to have with us
His sister Demetra, and his Aunt Loyce, And Niece
DeAnne besides our children and Grandchildren.

The Hope Center

You have read the testimony of Gesina Blaauw at the very beginning of my book. She is the little lady from Holland who was an early pioneer missionary to Albania. She had been in Albania since the walls of communism fell in that country. She had come to know our HFTW president, Jimmy Franks, through connections in European missions. He had invited her to America to speak about Albania in churches, and they had kept in close contact throughout the years as she began her official organization and mission work in Albania. She had purchased property in Marikaj, Albania, and converted it into a dormitory for handicapped people to be brought for physical therapy as well as for Christian teaching. Gesina has been a wonderful blessing in Albania for many years but felt God calling her to move a big portion of her ministry to the country of Africa. She still maintains a portion of property and a home adjacent to the original portion of land with two large buildings on it.

We heard about her wanting to sell her large property, so we went to talk with her about it. She said that it was worth every bit of, if not more than, $500,000. She proposed that price to us, but right away, we knew we did not have that kind of money. We came back home to the States and began to pray about it and talk with Jimmy Franks about her desire to sell this to us and how it would be perfect for what we were wanting to do. When we walked through it on our visit there in 2009, we had our pastor from Glen Haven and also our son-in-law, Andy Howard, with us. There were some other men with us, and we could see what a real need there would be to renovate the buildings. We would especially have to redo the largest three-story building before we could ever move any teens into that structure. It was in need of total rebuilding on the inside to make it into dorm-like rooms with a separate bathroom to go with each room. We wanted our facility to be something very nice for the kids and also a place to house guests who would come in from America at times to do work projects around the place. In order to do that renovation work, it was going to take most of the $200,000 we had set back and saved from the Night of Hope.

I remember at the time we were praying about Gesina's property, I was involved in a ladies Bible study at Glen Haven entitled "Believing God" written by Beth Moore. All through that study where I would write in my "Faith Journal," I was sharing the prayer request that God would somehow allow us to get that property from Gesina with just the $200,000 we had on hand. I also had all of the ladies "believing God" with me that he was going to answer this prayer and provide a way for us to get this property in a way that we could manage financially.

We contacted Jimmy Franks, founder of Hope for the World. Since he and Gesina had been friends from way back, at the beginning of our work in Albania, we felt he could help us. If Jimmy could convince Gesina to sell the property to us for $200,000 plus interest instead of $500,000, we might be able to make arrangements with her whereby we could pay her $50,000 up front with the balance in annual payments of $43,000 over the next four years, or a total of $222,000. Then we could do the renovations with most of the money we had at that time. Well, we bathed that proposal in much prayer. Jimmy contacted her and made the proposal. We knew this would help alleviate her immediate financial need and would also give her a substantial amount to look forward to receiving each year. We were so blessed that Gesina agreed, and in 2010, we took possession of what we now call "The Hope for the World Center" or, in the Albanian language, "Shpresa per Boten." This place has also become known throughout the country as "The Hope Center for Teens," where the teenaged orphans truly receive hope for their future.

We are so very thankful for the leadership of our Albanian president, Perparim Demcellari, who knew exactly who we needed to employ as the building contractor or, as they are called in Albania, the Engineer, who would be able to make the transformation to the property. Perparim has always done a superb job in making sure that we get the very most for our mission dollars in Albania. He worked together with the Engineer in drawing out the plans for the rooms in the three-story building. It would have one floor for the guys, one floor for the girls, and the very top floor would be made into two apartments, and there would also be room on that floor to make other sleeping rooms in the future.

And so the work began on those grounds. It was so exciting to see the progress and to be kept informed daily from Albania on how the work was going. Perparim was already going ahead and pricing custom-built bedroom furnishings for each room. We asked him to give us prices on what it would cost to completely furnish each bedroom which would sleep two teens. There were two single beds and a double closet that connected the two beds, one for each of the teens' personal use. There was also a very nice-sized bathroom with a walk-in shower, sink, toilet, and more cabinet space. When he gave us the total cost for furnishing each room in this beautiful facility, we began to put this need out in our newsletter and also to make it known to our Sunday school class at our church.

It was our plan to name each room for the person or family who furnished it completely. The total price for the bedrooms was $1,650. We were so blessed that practically all of those rooms were furnished by friends and families from our church. Others were furnished by our wonderful friends and supporters all around the country who were reading our newsletter monthly. It was truly amazing to see how these needs were supplied so that by the time we were ready to furnish the rooms, the money was all in hand. The beautiful plaque with the room sponsor's name was displayed just to the right side of the entrance to each bedroom. Inside the bedrooms, we also displayed a photograph of the person or family who provided the funds.

It has been a thrill to take some of these precious friends with us to Albania and let them visit our Hope Center and walk through and visit "their" room and see it being used daily by our young people. We also have a very special room near the balcony on the second floor where we have many, many photos of those who have contributed funds especially for this project. It is a huge board, and we call it our "Wall of Gratitude." The young people and any other visitors who come to our center can look at the faces and names of the many Christians who have cared and shared of their own hard-earned money. They have made a wonderful place for us to not only house but also train Albanian Christian young people to go out and make a difference in their society. Their own lives have been transformed through the grace of God, and they are ready and willing to give back the love and care they have received here.

We were blessed in our early years at the Hope Center to have a returning missionary, Pam Arney, on board. She had been a missionary in the early 2000s in Shkodra but had then returned to the States for a short time. God kept working on her to return to mission work, and even though she tried to look into other fields, God kept prodding her heart to return to Albania. She came to talk with us, and it so happened that we had an apartment she could live in, right there at our Hope Center. She is back in Albania, resides in the apartment on the property with the kids, and has been a huge blessing to them for many years now. She also introduced them to having a dog for a pet as she brought her own dog with her. At this particular time, she has increased her family to two dogs, and all of our teens love them so much and help her look after them whenever they are outside. The kids also have some cats who live on the property, and although our president, Perparim, has never before loved a cat or dog, one of the cats has truly wrapped him around her paw and made a best friend of him. It's funny how animals can worm their way into your heart.

The second apartment upstairs at the Hope Center belongs to Perparim and his wife, Aferdita. They actually have a home in Tirana, but they spend a lot of time there at Marikaj as well. It is such a beautiful country location, so quiet and cool that it makes a nice place for them to get away from the noise and activity of the capital city. Perparim and Aferdita are really in what would normally be termed their retirement years, but like us, as long as they can keep serving the Lord and taking care of the work he has given them to do with Hope for the World, they will do so. Both of their children and their grandchildren live in Canada and are employed there. There are many Albanians living in that country, as well as many living in Albanian settlements in the United States. Albanians are very smart and hardworking people.

This is truly a beautiful place on a wonderful piece of property in a small village between the airport and the capital city. It is a great location and has public schools close by that our kids attend. We have had it opened and have graduated kids for a number of years now. Most of the kids who have come through the Hope Center have also gone on to higher education or to specific vocational training to prepare them for their future. Every one of the kids has come to know Christ as their personal Savior and also has been discipled while living at the Hope Center. They have been trained in many ways through our staff. None of them knew anything but institutional living before they came to our Hope Center. At our place, we treat them as family. They live together as family. Each one has their own responsibilities in keeping the place very neat and clean. They learn how to manage their time and how to study as they have scheduled study hours daily under the leadership of our educator. They also learn many duties and chores that they never had been taught in any of the government institutions. The Bible is a vital and important part of their daily lives. They are also involved in helping evangelize the community through visitation, assisting the poor by bringing them food at times, and being actively involved in many youth activities held at the Hope Center for the community. Our center has truly become a hub of Christian activities for all ages, and we have seen a wonderful harvesting of souls in the area through our ministries there. To God be all the glory!

Our teens at the Hope Center are currently attending a church in Tirana on Sundays. We have seen many of our teens come to know Christ while residing at our Hope Center, if they came there without knowing him. If they had already come to Christ through Hope for the World's outreach in the various orphanages of Albania, the Hope Center has been a wonderful place for them to grow in Christ and learn the importance of following him in believer's baptism. We are happy to say that every one of our teens has been baptized and grown spiritually, as well as academically, by being a part of our HFTW family.

At the Hope Center, we have a wonderful staff of workers. One of them is Margarita who we came to know years ago when she was working in the Zyber Hallulli Orphanage. She was one of the first people we hired to be a part of our staff when we first started the Tag Center which was housed in the government building adjacent to the Tirana Zyber Hallulli Orphanage. Margarita is an educator and is very busy with our teens tutoring them and mentoring them to make sure they are ready to enter the University of Tirana or to further their education through some other specialized training in the country such as tourism, culinary school, journalism, and auto mechanics.

Since I have just mentioned Margarita, I want to mention that I have included in this book something from her that you will read later in our "Staff Testimonies." I was so blessed when I read what she had written.

It is our plan to establish a local church on our HFTW property soon. It may happen before this book is published. We are bringing in people of all ages, right on up to adults, for various Bible-centered functions and activities. They are coming faithfully to the center, especially other teens in the area. We have a great group of teens studying the Bible together every Tuesday night. We also have a huge group of children and teens coming every Saturday for Bible classes.

We have a wonderful staff in Albania working in all of the orphanages and staffing our Hope Center. They are all Albanian born, but best of all, they are born-again believers and love serving the Lord in the many different capacities for Hope for the World. In each and every orphanage where we are present, three in the city of Shkodra, one in Tirana, one in Korce, one in Saranda, and our Hope Center for Teens in Marikaj, our staff is able to tell them about Christ by having regularly scheduled Bible classes each week. We also have the opportunity to lead them in many extracurricular activities which are always God centered. We have also been free to bring the Gospel to the elderly at the center in Saranda.

I'd like to introduce you right now to my very close friend and our Missionary Mom at the Hope Center, who I have mentioned earlier on in my book. I asked Pam Arney to please put her testimony into a form that I could slip in between the covers of this *Albanian Attachment,* because if ever there was a lady who has had such a wonderful attachment to a country, it is Pam. Enjoy her testimony.

Pam Arney, Called By God

A life is defined by the events and choices from the moment of your first breath until the second of your last. My life began in 1963 when I entered the world as the youngest of seven children born into the Arney family. With that many kids in the house, daily life was an adventure. However, my true adventure began at age five when I accepted Christ as my personal Savior. At that time, I could never have imagined where God would lead me.

From my earliest memories, I was immersed in God's Word and life within the church. Having a father as a pastor tends to do that to you! Attending Christian schools and college made it easy to transition to teaching in a Christian school. Up to that point, missions wasn't even a blip on my radar. I enjoyed teaching and had a great group of friends to hang out with. Little did I know what was just around the corner.

In college, I fell in love with sign language and learned all I could. During my years of teaching, I incorporated it into my classroom in many ways. When the chance to join a mission team going to work at a deaf school in Jamaica came up, I jumped at the chance. This was my first taste of missions, but it would not be my last. Over the next couple of years, I made two more trips to Jamaica. Then God called me to leave the States and move to Jamaica as a teacher for the deaf. What a challenge it was to teach little children who had no language at all. The creativity God had blessed me with was stretched to find ways to help these little ones learn how to communicate.

After only a year and a half, God called me back to the States to help care for my parents. My mother was diagnosed with tuberculosis, and, as her health declined, we had to give her around-the-clock care. Mom went home to be with Jesus in March of 2000. Then my dad had to be put in a nursing home because of his health issues. Near the end of 2000, I could sense God was preparing me to return to the mission field, but where?

As I began to pray for direction, God opened the door for me to join a team going to Russia to visit orphanages. That was my first taste of being with orphans, but it would not be my last! When I returned to the States, I began searching for missions that had a focus on ministry to orphans. There were not a lot out there at the time. Every organization I looked at seemed to be a closed door. Then one day early in 2001, I was listening to the local Christian radio station. They were supporting a "Trek for Hope" fund-raiser. A man from Georgia, Fred Tag, was riding his bike from the coast of California to the coast of Georgia to raise funds for Hope for the World to build a place for the orphans in Albania to stay while attending high school. I knew nothing about Hope for the World and didn't even know where Albania was, but I sent in a donation and requested information about the organization.

Within a week, I received a packet of information in the mail from Roger and Cherie Mullins. What a surprise to find that they lived in the next town over from me. After praying about it, I set up an appointment to go by and visit them. They spent the evening sharing with me the work they were doing in Albania. We decided I would go for a month-long visit to see for myself if this was where God wanted me. In just a few weeks, God had provided the funds for me to go, and I was on my way to Shkoder, Albania, to stay with Prenda and Fredi Zefi.

I spent an awesome month loving on and holding the babies at the baby orphanage and playing with the children at the preschool and school-age orphanages. All during those weeks, I kept praying and asking God if this was where he wanted me and, if so, what in the world was I going to do?

About a week before I was to return to the States, I was praying, and God spoke so clearly to my heart that this was the place he had for me. I returned home at the beginning of March and immediately put my home on the market. I started making plans and raising the monthly support needed to live in Albania. My home was sold after only a month, and God brought in the funds so quickly that I was back in Albania by August 1, 2001.

The Hope for the World staff in Shkoder were such a blessing as I settled into life in Albania. Back then, the electrical power was off more often than it was on. Most days, we had no power until evening, and the power was so poor that you could only run one appliance at a time. "Do I cook dinner or wash clothes?" Decisions, decisions! Summers were very hot and winters were very cold, but what fun it was to see God working in our orphanages. Babies who before this time were months behind in development because of lack of human contact and stimulating activities began to catch up as Prenda and I spent time each day holding, talking to, and playing with them. We were able to start Bible classes in each of the orphanages, and we began to see the children coming to Christ. Soon, we had to start discipleship classes to help those saved grow in their walk with Jesus.

At the present time, I live and work at the Hope Center in Marikaj. Remember, I mentioned how I first heard about Hope for the World through the "Trek for Hope" fund-raiser? Well, the money raised allowed Hope for the World to renovate one of the buildings at the Tirana orphanage, and the teens were then able to stay there instead of having to move into the government dorms. The government dorms are a horrible place for orphans. They suffer a lot of abuse from the others who live there. Their things are stolen, and the girls are raped and beaten up by others because there is no one to protect them. Now, with the Tag Center, we could watch over them and provide for their physical and spiritual needs.

As things progressed, the Lord opened the door for Hope for the World to purchase property for a larger center. Each year, new students come to stay at the center with us. We are a family here, providing all that they need. My time is spent helping with homework, sewing and mending for them, encouraging them and teaching them basic ways to take care of themselves. Our goal for them is to give them a solid Biblical foundation and the necessary life skills to care for themselves when they leave the center. We have seen many come to Christ, but some have not made that decision yet. However, the seed is planted, and we trust God to continue to work out his plan in their lives as they step out of our doors and into the future plans he has for them.

As for me, God has given me a full life here. In addition to my work at the Hope Center, I have been blessed with the privilege of homeschooling two missionary kids and also working with Kids Clubs in Tirana and Marikaj. This is my earthly home now, and, if it is the Lord's will, I will continue to live and work here until he calls me home.

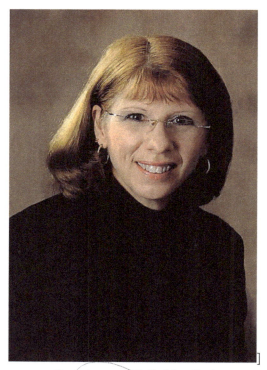

Pam Arney—Called by God
We are so blessed to have Pam working with
us at Hope for the World.

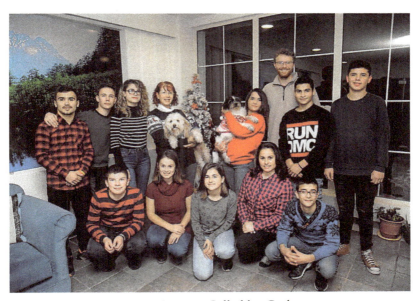

Pam Amey—Called by God
Pam and her two dogs, Nike and Sven Kids
from the Hope Center—2018

Activities at the Home Office

It has been my plan throughout my book to bring you back to the home base every now and then so you can see what our *Albanian Attachment* is like at home, right here in McDonough, Georgia. First of all, I'd like to give a big praise to our Lord and Savior for putting us in exactly the right house to be our home in McDonough. It was actually in 1996, when Roger was in Albania, that I found the home we are in now. We had been living in our rented townhouse apartment on Sentry Oak Court since December of 1990. We were blessed to live in a nice neighborhood and have really great neighbors in the adjacent apartment. It took us a number of years to sell our home in Virginia because it was more of a vacation home for people who just want to have a "getaway" place in the beautiful Blue Ridge Mountains. That was a long story, and I told all about that in my previous book subtitled *Joyous Journey*. After our home was sold, we had begun looking around Henry County, Georgia, to buy a place. A local realtor had shown us a number of places that were for sale but none to our liking. Either we would have to convert a bedroom into an office which would rob us of a guest room or it would have a bonus room upstairs which meant, as we were getting older, it would be difficult for us to climb the stairs many times a day. The houses we had seen just weren't matching up with our needs and desires.

However, when I entered this home in 42 East Subdivision in McDonough and saw the layout, I felt immediately in my heart of hearts. "You are home, girl!" The whole house was absolutely perfect for our needs. And it even had a well-constructed tree house and a chunky wooden playground in the backyard and a wooded area that would be great for our grandchildren! At that particular time, we only had Brady and Austin, and they were about seven and three years of age. I can remember writing an email over to Albania that day to one of our staff members. I told her to let Roger know that I had found a house for us! I think he may have thought that I was putting a down payment on it without him even seeing it, and I made sure he knew that was not so. At the time, I only knew the "asking price," and I had not made a counteroffer. I was going to wait until Roger came home in a few days to do that.

I never will forget the day Roger and I came to look at the house with our realtor to perhaps sign the contract. We had Brady and Austin with us who were, like I said, ages seven and three. Well, when they saw that tree house and the swings and slide in the backyard, they ran outside and then immediately came back inside and literally begged us to buy that house! By then, we were pretty well convinced ourselves, but I know that realtor was happy we had those boys along. She said that from then on, she would always insist that people bring their kids or grandkids along when she was showing a house!

Well, that was in the month of March of 1996, I believe. We had a few changes we wanted made inside the house that would take maybe two or three months to do. Our friend for many years, Brother Johnny Adkins, is an awesome carpenter and builder, so we hired him to do all of the changes inside the house. We thank God for him and his excellent work. So it was in June of 1996 when we actually moved into our home in McDonough. We have been at this address since that time, and it has suited our every need and been such a comfortable home not only for us to live in but also for entertaining. We have had so many of our wonderful Albanian family as well as our own immediate family and friends in the ministry visit with us here. We have three bedrooms and only use one for us, so we always have two guest rooms. Our offices are adjacent to the garage as you enter through the back doors. You also enter the kitchen from my office. This has been perfect for us when we have guests in our home. I can lay out their continental breakfast for them in the kitchen, and then they can get up and go in there any time they want. Roger and I can go right into the office to do any work we need to do and not bother any of our guests. They can have the whole house to themselves.

Since we have lived in this home, we have expanded our office area, as Roger was having to share the same office with me and Cindy, making it very difficult for all of us to work in one room. We called our friend, Brother Johnny, again, and he added two rooms onto the garage end of the front of the house. It hid the garage and gave us a room for our copier and file cabinets and another desk. Roger has his own private office just around the corner from that room. We really have a perfect setup here and plenty of room to take care of all of the office work connected with Hope for the World in Albania. Brother Johnny did a wonderful job making it look like it had been built that way. You can't even tell there was an add-on.

Our daughter, Cindy, has been working with us now for a good number of years. She works voluntarily, by her own choice. She does a beautiful job of communicating to the sponsors whenever we receive mail from their orphan in Albania. She also helps with so many of the bookkeeping tasks, and projects, that come up needing a special "touch." She is very gifted and loves her work, and she and I have an awesome time working together. I can't say we don't sneak off sometimes and do a "shopping" day. That is the joy of being your own boss and working voluntarily. No one can dock your pay. Ha ha.

Before Cindy came, we did have another wonderful secretary, Ann Blosfeld, who worked with us during a few of the earlier years. She helped us to get everything set up on our computers. She had the knowledge about databases, spread sheets, and various programs like Excel, Word, etc. I cannot tell you how much she taught me that made this work so much more organized and efficient than it was before she came. She was so good in fact that she got hired by a company that could really pay her what she was worth, so we had to let her go.

I will never forget how much fun we had here with Ann, though. She loved everything about our ministry. She had known us for years, so she knew of our music ministry with the family and was one of Buddy's biggest fans. She and her husband were members of our church at that time as well, so we shared all of that in common.

When she was here, she made what we called "The Office Bible." She put a notebook together with instructions on everything that we had set up in the office. This was so helpful to me through the years as long as we were using the same software.

Workdays were never really like workdays when Ann was around. We did a lot of work, but we always had so much fun in the middle of it. I believe God truly meant for her to work for us at that time. I hope she gets to read my book and reads this part and knows I mean every single word I am writing. She was "one in a million." I can remember one time when I needed my house really deep cleaned because we were going to be away in a meeting, and when we would be coming back, I would be having some of my special guests in our home. I had thought about hiring someone to do the work for me, and Ann volunteered. That was just the kind of friend and coworker she was! She did a tremendous job, and it looked so shining and bright everywhere when we got home. Well, this was a wonderful time while she worked for us. When I lost her, I tried one or two others to see if they could do the job, and I found it was really best for me to just work longer hours myself than to try to find someone as good as she was because I usually had to do the work all over again anyway whenever someone else did it.

This went on for a little while, and then Cindy, our daughter, had a change in their family business that allowed her time to come two or three days a week to help us. She has been voluntarily helping us ever since. We thank God for her every day.

You may wonder what there is to do that takes so much office work here at Hope for the World. Well, one of the first things we have tried to do is always keep our office very personally connected with those who are a part of helping us provide the funds for the ministry. We have a group of people that are known as "sponsors." That means they have chosen to personally sponsor at least one orphan in Albania at a cost of $30 per month. Over the months and years, there are many changes that take place in Albania. Some of the kids get adopted, some "age out" of the orphanage, and some of them have the good fortune to move back home with their family, if their family gets a stable income. Many of the children in Albania in the orphanages are there because of extreme poverty on the part of their families. Many others are there because parents have died or been killed in some type of tragic event. Others have been born out of wedlock and utterly abandoned and given over to the state. When changes take place in Albania as to the location of a sponsored child, it is Cindy's job to see that the sponsor knows that information and is given the opportunity to sponsor a different child to replace the one who has gone.

We started in 1994 with sponsorship of $30 per month, and we have not changed, even though the economy has changed over there, and it truly takes much more money now than it did when we first began our work. This has kept us really having to work hard to keep sponsors, as some will begin the program of sponsoring a child, and then they will get involved with something else or another mission and will drop their sponsorship. Then we have to find replacements for these sponsors. It is hard to say how much office time it takes when just one child has to be replaced for a sponsor. We have to notify the sponsor, make a selection, and then see if the sponsor is OK with that. If not, then we are back to the drawing board again, so to speak. Cindy handles 100 percent of the sponsorship program for us. She has also been a big part of posting the incoming checks and getting bank deposits ready. My particular job falls more in the lines of communicating back and forth with our staff in Albania. I'm also Roger's "secretary" which entails writing letters to our leadership over there, making decisions, planning upcoming projects, and planning for groups who go over to work in Albania. We also make travel arrangements for anyone, or any group, going over. We are in touch on a daily basis with our staff all over Albania. Now that we have Facebook messaging besides emails, it is done more quickly and efficiently. We can also have conferences using Skype, and it's like being right there in person with our staff. In just a matter of minutes, we can find who we are looking for if we need something in Albania or need to check on a child for their sponsor, etc. One of my other responsibilities has been to write our monthly newsletter. We have been putting out a family ministry newsletter ever since the beginning of our days in evangelism in 1977. Not a month has passed that we have not sent out a monthly newsletter. Let's see, that means we are approaching five hundred different newsletters through the years. Oh, my goodness! That's right, ever since 1977, we have had a mailing list and sent out a newsletter of some sort. Roger believes in keeping our people informed of what is going on in our work, and this has been our way to do this.

Some of Roger's duties in the office are staying in touch regularly with our staff in Albania. He is the one in charge of raising the funds for our monthly budget. He also sees to it that the funds are wired to Albania every month. In addition, he decides when we are going to have special fund-raising events for projects or for the physical needs of someone in an orphanage or on our staff in Albania. I guess you could say he is the "stress carrier" of the ministry. He not only has had the dreams for the ministry but has also had to design different ways we can implement to help carry out these dreams. Many wonderful projects in eight different facilities have been done in Albania since we began our "Albanian Attachment" in 1994.

Roger is also currently the errand runner on a daily basis which means trips to the post office, the bank, and the office supply store, bringing lunch sometimes, or taking us to lunch other times. He makes runs to the airport many times to pick up visitors from Albania or other places. He also opens all of the mail and sorts the checks into the categories for which they are intended before giving them to Cindy to post or to me to write a "thank you" note. He can always manage to keep both of us busy. During our entire ministry, Roger has been very careful to send thank you notes to people who help us in this ministry God has given us. He really would love me to write a thank you to every person who sends in a check for sponsorship each month, but we know that would be an impossible amount of letters and postage to mail them if we did so, plus it would be impossible for this poor secretary to find time to do that.

Roger has also been the "travel planner" for our trips in the ministry. He does all of our booking to mission conferences, getting the particulars together, and filling our calendar during the years we have been involved since 1994. One of his greatest gifts has always been encouraging others and thanking people personally for their support of our ministry. He does this naturally whenever he sees someone he recognizes as a sponsor or donor to Hope for the World Albania. Just in the past few months, due to his physical difficulties, arising from a stroke and a severe hearing loss, we have had to cut way back on our travels within the United States. Driving long distances has also become difficult the older we get.

There are some mission conferences and a very special Jubilee at Grand Strand Baptist Church in Myrtle Beach, South Carolina, that we still attend annually. We are grateful for the supporting churches that are so faithful to continue helping us financially each month with our ministry. If I could, I would write a lengthy portion about each and every church and pastor. They have all been such wonderful supporters to us and have made it possible for us to continue faithfully year after year. We still make our annual trip to Albania to meet personally with our staff as well as all of the children in the orphanages. While we are in the country, we also meet with the government directors of the state-owned orphan homes that we assist. We have developed a very strong bond and a good rapport with all of them. They are always very happy to see us. If Roger needs to attend any other meetings with members of the Albanian government while we are there, that is set up in advance prior to our visit each time. The part we love so much is loving on the orphans of all ages, the widows, and the elderly. But so very special is the time we get to spend with our precious staff who have been so faithful through the years.

I am including personal testimonies of our staff members whom we have been so privileged to have working with us in Albania. You have already read some of them. At this time, I would like to begin with a testimony from one of our secretaries, Anila Bushaj. This is a story that will not only touch your heart but will thrill you when you read what God has done in her life.

THE MAKING OF A WONDERFUL LIFE

Anila: A Love Story

I was taken to the Tag Center in December 1999. Before that, my sister and I used to live with our uncle's family in Albania. I was born in a nice city near the coast blessed by God with an amazing landscape and beaches. My father passed away when I was six years old and my sister was only four. My mother walked away, and we haven't seen her since then. My uncle made an oath to my father that whatever was going to happen, he was going to take care of me and my sister. And that's what happened. After my father's death, we moved to my uncle's house, which was in another town of Albania. My uncle and his wife had three children of their own who were older than my sister and I. We lived with them for about ten years. We never felt like a real part of that family as we weren't treated as part of it. I have had some very difficult moments in my life while living there, and this is when I turned to God. Before that, I had never heard about God, never heard the name of Jesus Christ. I was only nine years old when I first heard about Christ, I was so impressed by his love, grace, and mercy. I was eager to learn more, so I started studying about God and reading the Bible by myself without any guidance, and I was filled with love. This was a love that I never felt before. It was a feeling of immense love, joy, hope, peace, and protection. For the first time in my life, I didn't feel alone, I actually felt very blessed.

A few years later, when I was a young teenager, my uncle could not care for us any longer due to financial problems. I was actually happy to be leaving that place. So I and my sister were taken to orphanages; I was taken to the Tag Center, operated by Hope for the World (HFTW) for teens only, and Klea was taken to the Tirana Orphanage because of her being younger than I. These buildings were adjacent to one another, so I was still close enough to see her every day, and this was comforting to both of us.

Living at the HFTW teen center, for the first time in my life, I felt at home. I loved it even more when I heard about this Jesus

Christ whom I have been trying to find all my life, as he was the one I read about in the Bible and the one who filled my life with joy. At that time, I wasn't saved and had not yet heard about salvation. But one day, my roommate at the Tag Center shared with me about salvation, and that day, I accepted Christ as my Savior and the ruler of my life. That was the happiest day of my life. Then I understood that my relationship with Christ was eternal and that I was finally set free. I was cleansed from sin, free of anger, fear, and desperation, and I now had a hope for my future.

I spent the best four years of my life at the Tag Center, as my faith was getting stronger, and I was being discipled in Christ. I knew little about what God was preparing for my journey ahead, but I was anxious to know. I graduated from high school in 2002, and at the same time, I was taking some English classes which had been provided for me by HFTW. Taking these classes turned out to be very significant in my life. I also received much advice and wise counsel from Perparim Demcellari, who was our HFTW Albanian president as well as the director of the teen center.

After graduating from high school, I went to the Tirana University to study for social work. I felt God's presence in my life. While in college, through HFTW and the generosity of the staff, I was hired by HFTW in Tirana as the secretary for the Albanian president of HFTW. During this time, I got a chance to share some of the love of God with other orphan children at the orphanage through Bible classes as well. I was so happy to have the opportunity to share about the greatest love of all, the love of Christ who died for us when we still were sinners, and how through his death on the cross he washed away our sins and cleansed us. I taught them that all they needed to do to be forgiven and experience this great salvation was to pray and accept Jesus.

It is amazing how God's love can turn things around and turn your trials into a triumph. I worked with HFTW for about eight years, until one day, my dear friend, who at that time was my boss, Cherie Mullins, told me about this nice Christian guy in the state of Kentucky, who wanted to chat with me and to get to know me better. Brother Roger Mullins happened to know this guy's father ever since they were both teenagers. It was Jesus Christ who brought them together. I'll let Cherie tell you something about their relationship.

Editor's Note: It's a real joy and privilege to tell you how amazing our God is and how he alone can bring things to pass that we could never imagine. As Anila mentioned, when Roger was a teenager and a member of Oak Grove Baptist Church in Moore's Chapel, Tennessee, one Sunday, which was designated as "Youth Sunday," they had a special guest speaker at the church who was also a teenager, just a few years older than Roger. His name was Jerry Horner, and he was a Bible college student from Union University in Jackson, Tennessee. He gave the message on that Sunday morning, and Roger was sitting on the back row of the church with his cousin, Butch, and some other friends. He said he wasn't really paying a lot of attention to the sermon, but it seems that when Jerry Horner gave the invitation that day, the Holy Spirit really spoke to Roger about his need to be saved. He went down the aisle and landed on his knees at the altar where Jerry Horner met him and led him to Christ. Roger was fifteen, and Jerry was eighteen at that time.

Through Jerry's friendship with Roger's family, he got to know him well, and actually through all of the years, there has been a connection so that we knew of the various ministries in which Jerry has been affiliated. He is now Dr. Jerry Horner. He was a professor at Oral Roberts University for a number of years. At the present time, he still teaches Bible seminars nationally and internationally. He is still traveling extensively even though he is in his eighties.

As it happened, one time in the spring of 2013, when I was writing our monthly newsletter, I included on the front page an article about Anila. I had a very pretty picture of her posted in the article, and I just casually mentioned, "By the way, Anila is still single."

Well, a short while after that newsletter went out, we had a phone call from Dr. Jerry Horner. He was coming to Atlanta on some business and would be coming close to our home. He wondered if he could drop by for a visit. We were delighted and told him to definitely plan to stop by. I baked an angel food cake with fresh strawberries and whipped cream for the occasion. We hadn't seen Jerry in a year or more. When he came that day, I left him and Roger alone in the living room visiting for some time before I went in to join them.

When I sat down, Brother Jerry said to me, "Cherie, I noticed an article in your recent newsletter about a young lady named Anila."

I said, "Yes."

And he then asked me if I thought she would be at all interested in meeting a nice Christian young man. It turned out he was speaking of his son, Thad. Thad was about thirty years of age at that time and had never found Mrs. Thad Horner yet but was open to trying to get acquainted with Anila if she was open to communicating with him through Facebook. Anila was about twenty-eight years of age at that time, and I felt like she would be really excited to know that a young Christian American man was wanting to get acquainted with her. So I told Dr. Horner that I would ask her and then get back with him. I did, she was thrilled, and so it began.

I met Thad Horner in June of 2013. It was through HFTW, and through my special friend, Mrs. Cherie Mullins, who wrote the article about me in the newsletter. I can never thank her enough for that. I thank God for bringing her and Brother Roger and HFTW into my life. I thank Jesus for the man he found for me. *Only his plan is the best, and it always works and never fails.* So first it was the online chatting for about four months, and during that time, we found out that we were perfectly suited for one another. Then, in September of 2013, Thad came to my country, Albania, and we met for the first time in person. He spent eight days there. During this time, we got to know each other better, and we fell in love. We spent a lot of time together. We went to different places in Albania, so he got to know more about my country, its history, culture, etc. We loved our time together, and this is when I became his serious girlfriend, for real.

After he left, we continued to stay in touch, through the chatting. We would chat each day, and our love was growing for one another. Then, in December, he came to Rome, and I met him there, and we became engaged on his first day there at the beautiful Trevi Fountain in Rome, a very romantic place. That was the most amazing moment of my life when Thad proposed to me. We got to spend the Christmas holidays together there in Rome, and it was my very first time to be there as well as his first time. We got to know more about each other, and for me, it was the best Christmas ever. We had a blast!

We parted ways again. He went back to America, and I went back to Albania, but I was engaged now, and I had to begin the process of obtaining a "fiancee visa" in my country before I could ever come to America to be married to Thad. We began it as soon as possible, and we stayed doing our communicating online for about a year, and, finally, after all the struggles we went through concerning the documents, and after all the waiting, I was able to come to the United States in December of 2014. We were married on December 21, 2014 (near the day of Christ's birth). We have been married ever since then, and I am so blessed. God has opened many doors for me. Thad was a part of the staff at Asbury Theological Seminary in Louisville, Kentucky, where we first lived. We are now making a move to Tulsa, Oklahoma, as Thad has a new position with Oral Roberts University.

I am now able to have a job in America, so I am busy working every day. Before I had my papers and was approved to be able to work, I volunteered my services with Nightlight Christian Adoption Services. It was a blessing to get to know them, and during the time I worked there, doing voluntary work, we were able to accompany their administrator to Albania to help get them approved to handle Albanian adoptions. This has been approved now, and there are already families adopting from Albania. I am so blessed by this.

God has also blessed me with a wonderful family. I love Thad's parents like they were my very own, actually better than I ever loved my own because I didn't know them much. We have wonderful Christian friends, and I teach a Bible class to children at a local church in Nicholasville, Kentucky. I love doing that. It is important to teach the new generation about Christ and his importance in our lives. I want to do all I can for his kingdom. God has a great plan for each one of us, and I am so happy for his leading in my life and that I am a part of this global Christian family.

With love in Christ, Anila.

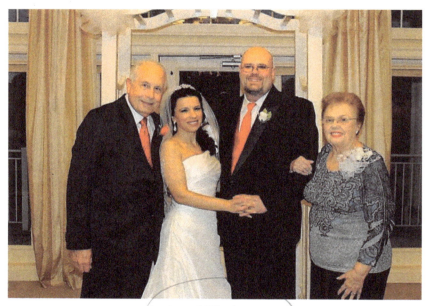

Anila and Thad Horner
Thad's Parents, Dr. and Mrs. Jerry Horner

Cindy's Comments

> For God so loved the world that He gave His only and beloved son Jesus Christ, so that everyone who believes in Him will not perish, but have eternal life. (John 3:16)

Mom asked me to write a little something to put in her book describing the work of HFTW Albania from my perspective and to share my small part of what I get to do in the ministry of HFTW.

I really did not know how to start, so I will start here, 1994.

This was the year Dad felt the leading of the Lord for him and Mom to turn their ministry focus from gospel music and evangelism to foreign missions. For as long as I can remember, my parents have been in some kind of Christian service and/or employment. When I was a young girl (first grade), my dad felt the call to preach. From that time forward, he and Mom have served on church staffs, singing in gospel groups and traipsing all over the country in evangelism with us kids! It was not a surprise at all to me that God was now turning their hearts toward this work, this country, and this ministry. They have literally been missionaries in their own right to many people through the years here on US soil. I have watched as they have mentored and ministered to countless people they've come in contact with over the years that were not even directly connected to their current job description. I guess you could say they are missionaries at heart and always have been. Now, the Lord had opened a new door for them to really focus on helping and ministering to Albanian orphans, and it sounded both exciting and a little scary, I must confess. But from day one, they knew this was what God would have them do, and they set about it, and here we are many years later, and this book is just a small account of what the Lord has done through a couple (in their fifties at the time) when they stepped out on faith and followed his new calling. I have been both a spectator and a very enthusiastic participant, so where I'm able, in support of this ministry, I will elaborate a little.

During the first years of their mission, I worked alongside my husband, Andy, at a company he managed and then owned. I was blessed to be able to work hours that let me be home when our children got home from school. This was the case from 1995 to 2006. I would help Mom monthly with doing the newsletter and other light office work I could do in my spare time. In 2007, Andy went to work for another company, and I went to work for HFTW on a regular basis. I can say that the past ten years have been the most rewarding for me as I have had the opportunity to work in their home office a few days a week in the area of sponsorship coordination and bookkeeping. This is truly a labor of love for me, and I am thankful and grateful to the Lord for allowing me to get to spend time working with them and for the staff of HFTW Albania.

My first trip over to Albania was in 2005 when I went with a small group from our home church, Glen Haven Baptist. I am not sure what I expected when I got there, but it surpassed anything I could have ever imagined. At that time, Mom and Dad had been involved in Albania for eleven years. I, like everyone else, had seen photos and videos of the horrendous state of the orphanages and the country in the beginning years. To go over there and see how much God had done in these orphanages and with the children throughout those years with the outpouring of love from the churches and individuals here in America was overwhelming. Of course, these orphanages were still institutions, not homes. The love we felt and saw displayed from the HFTW staff to these children was unbelievable as well as their love shown back to us. I have seen and felt so much appreciation from the people in Albania for what HFTW and all of the staff were doing for those children. This trip changed my life in so many ways. I first of all got to see how the Lord had used my parents' obedience to affect and change lives, but also I got to meet the talented godly staff members the Lord had provided in Albania to carry out the work.

In a way, I fell in love with the country and people of Albania in 2005. I understood now, firsthand, why Dad came back in 1994 and told Mom, "We have to go. We have to help them." I fully understood now.

I am not sure I expected Albania to be so beautiful. Never really spending any time in a European country before, I had not experienced the majestic beauty of the landscape of the mountains next to the sea and the breathtaking views like I saw that year. Of course, it was such an odd contrast to the plight and poverty of the people there who mostly had been living in utter destitution for years. The extreme contrast of these precious children living in this beautiful country in such horrendous conditions was heartbreaking to say the least. Our group visited all of the orphanages HFTW was involved in at that time. We traveled from the north of Albania to the very southern city of Saranda. We got to do a little bit of sightseeing and visit some of their historical sites while there, like the ancient cities of Butrint, Kruja, and Durress, and some medieval castles. Again, I was overwhelmed by the age of this country and to realize that their ancient history goes back to the days of Christ and the apostles. And as you have read in this book in the early chapters, places where Paul and Peter and Titus had been on missionary journeys.

In 2009, I was privileged to go back to Albania and this time with my husband and my son, Austin, who was fifteen at the time. We were with another group from our home church, and we were able to once again visit the children in the orphanages and the teens at the Tag Center. My husband, Andy, was one of the men who went to view the potential new property in Marikaj that Dad and HFTW were looking at to become our own administrative headquarters and Hope Center for HFTW Albania. That was an exciting trip, and it was wonderful to experience it with my family. Our older son, Brady, had already been to Albania three times. He went first with my parents and once with a group from another local church in our area. Later, as pastor of student ministries, he took a group of teens to Albania for a work project. So now, all of our family had been there and experienced Albania and the work being done by HFTW.

I must mention that through these visits, my heart had become entwined with the Albanian staff members there who I dealt with on a weekly basis through emails concerning sponsorship of the children, etc. However, while I was in Albania, we became more than coworkers, we became family. To this day, some of my closest extended family are my Albanian family. This is another blessing that I could have truly never expected. Such a blessing how God brought these precious people into our lives and through our mutual love for the Lord knit our hearts together as one big family.

In 2016. I was able to go back to Albania with my parents (just us three this time), and I got to spend some quality time with my Albanian sister, Prenda Zefi, and her family. What a special time this was as I actually got to spend a couple of nights in her home and be with her beautiful family, husband, Fredi, children, Edona, Tedi, and Reuel, and recent foster child, Klodjan. It is amazing how the Lord can put lives together when we live so far apart. But it's all through a shared love of Christ and our ministry ties.

I have also grown close to other members of our Albanian staff there. In Shkodra, there is Mirela Ymeraj, who was HFTW's first Albanian employee who I love like a sister. Fatos and Mirela Demiri, in Saranda, lead the work there in the orphanage as well as the elderly center known as Threshold of Hope. Ledina, our wonderful young woman who works so hard in the office headquarters for our in-country president, Perparim, and his wife, Aferdita. All of these staff members have come to America to visit in my parents' home, and it has bonded our friendship even more. I also have come to know other staff members who have been such a blessing to us while there. Nikolin and his beautiful wife, Nirvana, Sokrat and Tuku, Margarita, Albana, Teuta, and all the ladies who work at the Hope Center for Teens. The Lord has put together such a wonderful Albanian team for HFTW, and it is an added bonus that they feel like members of our family. How great is our *God*? He's good, so good, and he proves it over and over to me in so many ways.

A highlight of our trip in 2016, Mom and I had the privilege to minister alongside each other at a ladies meeting at Fredi and Prenda Zefi's home church, Bible Baptist Church, in Shkoder, Albania. This was one of the most awesome things I'd ever gotten to be a part of. Their pastor's wife, Linda, and the ladies of the church had organized a beautiful night for women in the community to come to the church for food and fellowship. Mom played the piano that night and I sang, and then my mom shared with the ladies on the theme of "A Legacy of Love." There were over seventy ladies there in attendance that night. Many were unsaved from the community, many were widows, many were ladies from the church, but all shared the common bond of being daughters, women, moms, and grandmothers. We were both so thrilled to get to be a part of something so very special. Mom shared her Christian upbringing and how important it is to know the Lord and bring your family to know him. She presented the Gospel as well to just add some water to the seeds that were being sown there in Shkodra by the Christians.

After the service, we were invited to spend some time with the young married ladies of the church in an "afterglow"-type setting at one of their homes. They wanted to have a time to ask Mom and I about what it looks like to have a "Christian home and a Christian marriage." They were raising children and wanted to have some encouragement on how to keep them involved in the church as they grow up. You see, they are some of the very "first fruits" of Christianity since their country had been steeped in communism and atheism for nearly fifty years from 1947 to 1992. They did not come from Christian homes, they are all basically new in the faith and have no examples of Christian leadership to look to for this type of guidance.

While I felt completely unworthy and ill-equipped to answer their questions, we still tried to be open and honest and share with them all we could in that small amount of time. We now have a whole new bunch of little sisters in the Lord in that Albanian town of Shkoder. I will never forget and always love and pray for them.

Some of us have become better friends since then through social media, although we don't speak the same language! Pictures are not language specific, thank goodness! And neither is *love*! It works in any language!

Another way I have been able to grow close to our Albanian staff and friends is by my favorite pastime and hobby known as "shopping." On many occasions, when any of our Albanian ladies has been here in the States visiting Mom and Dad, I have had the joy of taking them out to do some shopping! Sometimes it has been their first time to even visit our country, so a very exciting thing for them to do in the United States! How fun is this! Honestly, it's the best "perk" of my job at HFTW, I'm just trying to figure out how to somehow work it into a more full-time role! Ha ha! Honestly, I have loved this aspect of connecting with my Albanian family and friends. Women are all alike no matter what country we are from, we can all find a connection over a beautiful handbag or some killer shoes and some super sales! ☺

Working for Hope for the World Albania in our home office in Georgia is a joy and a privilege. My parents seem to enjoy it, too, because it insures a visit from their daughter on a regular basis! Even though we live just twenty minutes apart, and go to the same church, you can imagine that the busy schedules we all carry with our families and church family can pose quite a problem when it comes to just drop-by visits. So my working with them lets us attack two birds with that proverbial stone, so to speak.

Part of my busy time is spent babysitting my second grandchild, Adaline Grace Howard, who was born on August 31, 2017. She is little sister to Beau Andrew Howard who was born on April 3, 2015, and is already in a day care center where his mommy teaches school each day.

I love my Lord, my family, my church, and my work for HFTW Albania. I love the quotation that hangs on the walls of our office by John Wesley that says:

> *Do all the good you can by all the means you can.*
> *In all the ways you can. In all the places you can.*
> *At all the times you can. To all the people you can,*
> *As long as ever you can.*

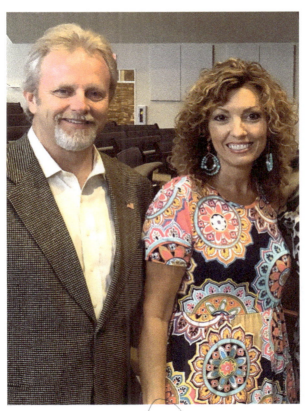

Andy and Cindy Howard
We are blessed to have Andy as a son-in-law.

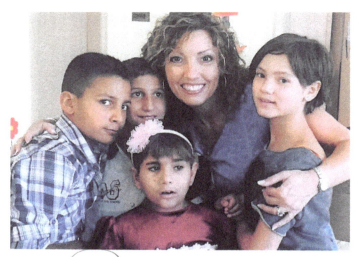

Cindy on one of her trips to Albania.
She loves these kids and they love her too!
She knows their names from working in the office.

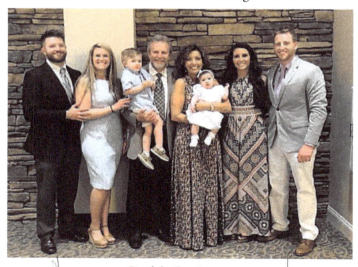

Cindy's Comments
Whole Howard family…
Cindy and Andy holding the grandchildren,
Beau and Adaline On the left are Brady and Savannah—parents
of the two grands. On the right are Austin and Suzanne-
Brothers married sisters… Very special!

Staff Testimonies

Margarita Gjoni

Before I became a staff member of Hope for the World, I had been a high school teacher in Tirana for seventeen years. I began working for Hope for the World in 1998 when they needed someone as an educator and administrative associate in the teen center that became first to be known as the Tag Center in Tirana and now as the Hope for the World Center, or just Hope Center for Teens, as we sometimes call it. I became a Christian in 1999.

The Lord has used Hope for the World to change my life, by giving me a bigger heart and a humble attitude. It seems to me that I had been focused on two things in life. First, to take care of my family, and secondly, to help the orphans. That is where the world would start and end for me. However, many things have changed for me since we began having the Kids Bible Club in Marikaj, bringing in children from the community who were not orphans. A lot of things have changed in my thinking. I feel that I must stay with and help these children too, even though they are not orphans. I can't stay without helping if I know how to do something that is needed. My heart really hurts as I see the kids of this community who actually have parents, but in reality, they act like they do not. I would see how rebellious they would act and how aggressive they were when we first started the Kids Bible Club.

This program of weekly Kids Bible Club, as well as teenage Bible Study each Tuesday evening, has connected us more with the community and has made all of our hearts softer. Having the kids from the community with us several times during the week has helped us to know the parents of these kids. I really feel honored and blessed now when a parent comes from the village and asks me if I can go to the school and represent them today because their child has caused problems and they will be working in the field so they cannot go to the school. I am able to do this at times, and I count it a privilege to do so.

When we first started the Kids Bible Club, some of the parents would not even allow their kids to come. However, today, when they see any of us walking around Marikaj, shopping or doing other things, they will come and talk with us with so much respect. I am blessed when I hear some of them tell me, "I know how my son is, so if he causes you any problem, don't hesitate to come and let me know as I know how to take care of this." They have confidence in us.

I really feel we do have the distinct privilege of sharing the gospel here in Marikaj and to be the light in a dark place where 100 percent are Muslim.

Another great blessing I have had lately during my work as a staff member at the Hope Center in Marikaj has been the special meetings we have held for the ladies and teachers of the community. At first, when we began inviting them to our center for special occasions, they would accept the invitation just out of respect to us. But now, they will always come whenever we have something special going on here, for example, for Christmas and Easter, when we have special services and invite the community.

After one of the teachers heard the message from our resident missionary, Pam Arney, recently for Mother's Day. She said: "Now I understand why your teens are so much different and special in school. They not only have you, the Hope for the World Staff, but they also have the Lord." How thrilling to hear her acknowledge that truth.

I am the educator (teacher) here at the Hope Center for Teens, among other things. I am really blessed that the teens who have graduated from high school and left the Hope Center are on their way in their adult lives. Eighty-five percent of them have finished the university, and a good number of them now have their own families and their own jobs. Hope for the World has done for them what a healthy biological family should do, and I am so honored to be a part of this great ministry.

Teuta Korra

I grew up in the orphanages in Albania. During the time I was living at what was known as the vocational school in Tirana, Hope for the World was providing 100 percent of all the needs because the government's economic situation during that time was so bad. It was easy for me to want to know the Lord because of the lives of all of the missionaries who came to share the love of Christ with us. I believe that their love and care for us as orphans led us to believe in God and to love the Lord.

I know at my young age, before I really fully understood, I prayed to accept Jesus several times because I wasn't sure. However, when I became a teenager, it was at that time that I got down on my knees at our Tag Center in Tirana and accepted Jesus as my Lord and Savior.

My biological family began to show interest in me once more. First, they thought that I would never forgive them for leaving me in the orphanage and keeping other siblings at home, but because of Hope for the World, there wasn't a thing I felt I was missing in my life, and I never got angry or mad at them. Hope for the World has given me all that a family could give me.

It was later, after I had left the orphanage, that God truly blessed my life and allowed me to go to work for Hope for the World, first as a dorm monitor, and now I have many responsibilities with the kids at the Hope Center. I now have ten kids I oversee daily and stay with them during the night. If any of them is sick, I am there to help them, day or night. I also make sure all of them get ready for school each day. I also enter into all of the activities at the Hope Center that we conduct for our own teens as well as events that include kids from the community. The Lord has not yet allowed me to be married or be a mom, but he has blessed me beyond measure by the work he has given me to do with Hope for the World.

What I really love is that I get to go home to see my biological family once a week, and the next day when I return to the Hope Center, I am greeted by our youngest siblings, who are twins, Arlind and Megisa. They come running to me and hug me and tell me how much they have missed me. That truly makes my life very happy!

Albana Lika

Albana Lika graduated from a professional school for teaching in 1990. She has been both a supervisor and a teacher in elementary schools. From 1990 to 1997, she has worked as an educator at the school-age orphanage, "Zyber Hallulli" in Tirana, Albania. She loved her job as a teacher of the children, and because of this reason, we are so happy to have her on our staff at the Hope for the World Center. She is using her gifts in helping our teens prepare for their future and also helps as a general assistant in the kitchen when needed.

Since coming to Hope for the World, she has grown as a Christian and believes in God with her whole heart and knows that through him, her life has been changed. We are blessed to have Albana as a part of our Hope for the World family.

Working with orphans every day sometimes makes me see it just as a job. But at the end of their time spent with us at the Hope Center, when we see that they have truly become really good young men and young ladies, my heart gets touched. I then realize what a great privilege I have been given to work here and to see the big changes in their lives and to know that God is the one who has done this. Truly, they are not orphans at all as God has taken care of them even more than any of their biological families have ever cared for them. Many of them had been totally abandoned or rejected by their own families, and that is why they were raised in the orphan homes.

I am ready to do anything that God has called me to do here at the Hope Center. He has used me to be involved in this ministry to the kids, but he has also changed my own heart. He has helped me to be a better person. When we first began to have the Kids Bible Club in Marikaj and invited the community kids to attend, I saw so many kids who weren't able to control themselves. They seemed to be in a war they were fighting. I sometimes had a lot of questions in my mind, *Am I in the right place? Can I handle all of this?* Now I definitely have to say I am ashamed that I even thought that way. I now love the Saturday morning Kids Bible Club, and it seems like all of these kids come here and really make this property feel alive. God is great!

One of my favorite moments here at the Hope Center with our teens is when they leave in the morning to go to school. They will hug me and they will ask, "What are we going to have for lunch today?" Or as soon as they finish lunch, they will ask me, "So what do you have for us for dinner?" We are all like one big happy family here, and I feel so blessed.

I got saved years ago at the International Church in Tirana. At first, I only attended because people were kind and invited me to come. After listening to the messages, I truly believed what I was hearing was from God's Word, and I gave my heart to Jesus. I will never regret that day. He blesses my life more and more as I live for him.

Personal note from Cherie: Albana is a part of all that goes on in our ministry at The Hope Center and even helps sometimes at the orphanage in Tirana. What a sweet servant's heart she has, and we are so blessed she is a part of our staff.

She's a great cook, too! We get to experience that each time we go to the Hope Center in Marikaj.

CHERIE Y. MULLINS

Nikolin Lekaj

I was born on 1940 in Albania.

I studied biochemistry at the University of Tirana. I have worked as a teacher for forty years, thirty-four years in different villages and six years as a school director in town. I retired in September 1997. In 1999, I started working with HFTW. The reference for my hire to Mr. Roger was from my school friend who has passed away, Memtaz Hafizi, who was then the HFTW Albanian director.

My duties while working for HFTW:

Purchased food and clothing

Assisted in the celebration of seven different feasts (holidays) during the year

Organized excursions with the kids

Organized summer vacations for the kids

Supervised different construction projects in four institutions

These projects consisted of reconstruction of the buildings, plastering, painting, laying tiles, installing new water systems, heating systems, playgrounds, building a greenhouse and setting up gardening, etc. The expenses for these projects have been very high. Just at the preschool orphanage, every year, I have spent $6000–$12000. I am very thankful to Mr. Roger and Mrs. Cherie that they hired me in the most needed time of my life. The job with HFTW was totally new for me but at the same time a real pleasure. Through the money that Roger and Cherie raised through sponsorship and other fund-raising projects, many orphans of our country have been helped. HFTW brought some missionaries that had a vision for the life, for the work, and for the friendship, which was a new thing for us who were very isolated. From these good believers, we have learned a lot from their wonderful humanitarianism and love.

HFTW gave us the chance to visit the United States and to know a different world and culture. In my family circle, I have made known the job that HFTW does and as for what I am in debt to Roger and Cherie. I will not forget even a single day, as long as I live, and I'll pray to Jesus Christ for them and that always I will have a thankful heart toward them. I was blessed to be retired from HFTW in the summer of 2017 after eighteen years of service.

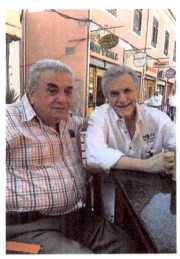

Nikolin was hired after he retired as a public school teacher In Albania. He has been like a wonderful Grandfather "Gjyshi" To all of the children in the orphanages in Shkoder.

Ledina's Story

This first part is from the letter we received from Ledina right after she had been hired by Perparim Demcellari to replace Anila Bushaj as our HFTW Secretary in the Tirana and Marikaj office in 2014. This is quite lengthy, but Ledina has proven to be a real answer to our prayers in so many ways. She came to us with much experience in the corporate world and also as a mature Christian young woman. I believe she has a lot to say that will be a blessing and will also shed light on the work of our ministry at The Hope Center in Marikaj, where she has been a very strong leader administratively as well as spiritually.

My name is Ledina Rabdishta, and I am twenty-nine years old as I write this. God has blessed me by allowing me to be a part of the foundation, Hope for the World, in Tirana, Albania. I want to thank you from my heart for the wonderful opportunity you have given me to be able to have a job in the Lord's work with Hope for the World.

My family took my sister and me to the New Hope Baptist Church in the Kinostudio area of Tirana when we were in the first grade of school. I have continued to go to that church even though my family members were not Christians. After being in many services and hearing God's Word, I opened my heart and invited Christ in as my Savior when I was ten years old. Then it was three years later that I got baptized. I praised God then, and I still do today that Christ died on the cross for my sins. I am very thankful for everything he has done, and still does, for me. I am still a member of New Hope Baptist Church where I try to be faithful with my attendance and service for God.

I have enjoyed a good period of growth in my church since I was a kid through the children's meetings and later in youth group, camp, and other activities. I have also been part of different discipleship classes. God kept working with me, and for some time, I have been the teacher of the fourth grade in Sunday school. In all of this, I have experienced great blessings from God and have also been encouraged and blessed by many others in our church who serve him faithfully.

During the years that I have attended church, I had my grandparents coming to the church to support me in different activities in which I was involved, like Christmas or Easter dramas and choir musicals. Later on, they were being a little more faithful in attending the regular church services. My parents usually come to church for special services. My mother is saved, and I am praying for my father to make a public profession of his faith in our Lord Jesus Christ as his personal Savior.

In my professional life, I have a Bachelor's Degree in Social Science and a Master's Degree in Communications. Since I was nineteen years old, I have been working for a film company in Tirana where, in the last six years, I have had a job as personnel supervisor of employees of the film company. I have done many different things and trained in Albania and abroad on the professional aspect of my job. Because Cherie has asked, I am now going to include a part in my testimony as to just how I got that job with the film company and some particulars connected therewith.

After graduating from high school, my sister, Eni, and I were looking for a job. Eni and I are just one year apart and have grown up more like twin sisters than anything else. We have lived our lives together, sharing the same bedroom in our small home, etc. It is very hard for students to get a job in Albania, a summer job, or a part-time job.

Our mom was working in an area near what is known as the Stephen Center, and she was asking everyone she met if they could find a job for us. One day, one of her neighbors asked her, "Do they know how to do anything?"

My mom answered, "They speak English, Italian, and some French. Please, if you have a job for them, let me know. I just want them to get used to working, even if they don't get paid." So she told my mom to tell us to come and meet her at the Film Company Studio (which was only two minutes from our home). We met her, and we got the first DVD to translate. We were so excited that we had a job, and we didn't even ask how much money we were going to get paid. In ten days, we sent them the translation of the movie. They liked it, and they gave us the next one and the next one and then the next one. So for six months, they didn't pay us because my Mom told them she just wanted her daughters to work.

On December 31, 2005, they called us and wanted to see us urgently. We were both so scared of what was going to happen. Why did they want to meet us? The owner of the company said, "I need this movie translated in two days, and you *will* get paid for it. Can you do it?"

We were so excited, and we said yes immediately. We didn't ask her how much she would pay us, but when we were leaving the company, we asked the security guard if he had any idea how much they paid translators for one day. He said he thought eight dollars. We were happy with that! Because of lack of electricity in our home, we had to work at an Internet café. It wasn't comfortable at all, but we finished the movie on time. We sent the translation the next morning at eight o'clock. The owner of the company was very happy, so she sat with us and said we would get paid for our job. One movie was $40. We were shocked because our parents earned only $10 per day!

We continued to translate, and they prepared an office for us. Man! We started to feel that we had a real job. During school hours, we would work four hours a day. They started to trust us with larger responsibilities. We could suggest other translators to them, and so many friends from our church began to get work for the company, and some of them still work for them even now.

When I earned my bachelor's degree, they offered me the job as personnel director of the company. The master's degree program I had applied for was from five to nine each evening, so I accepted the offer and started to work full-time. I was the youngest employee, so at the beginning, it was difficult to gain the respect from other employees. I was very strict about the work but also respected them at the same time. Soon everyone started to accept me and help me. We became good friends. My sister, Eni, was also promoted in her work as a translator and contact person for companies from all over the world where we were buying movies.

At this point, we could suggest movies to the board of directors. We had heard about a series of children's movies with Christian themes, such as *Veggie Tales*, *Charlie Brown*, *Super Book*, and other movies that told stories from the Bible. Sometimes, they would find them boring compared to *Mickey Mouse*, or other Disney productions, but I would always find a good reason why these movies had to be dubbed into Albanian, too. I wanted to show them at the right time on TV, at the peak time such as Christmas Day or Easter.

I also created a project, "Around Us," where I wrote the theme song, and the puppets I chose had "Jesus Loves Me" and "God Loves Me" written on their shirts. I was blessed as I had a chance, through God's direction, to employ many people from our church and even kids who still do the voices. God has used me in many ways, and for this, I am really thankful! I was very happy that so many of my brothers and sisters in Christ were also working at the Film Company. Everyone at the Film Company noticed a different attitude in their daily work and in the way that they would face difficult situations. Lots of people began to see Christ in our lives, and so many came to visit our church. Some even were saved, and a couple of teens came to the youth camp; one of them was the son of my boss. The Film Company has provided some things for the youth camps such as puppets, life-sized animal costumes for us to wear, and movies dubbed into Albanian. They are a real blessing and help to our ministry in Marikaj.

God has been so good to us, and he has taught us great lessons through giving to others. During Christmas, we decided to support the Sunday school classes for kids with refreshments and snacks at the churches in Tirana and in Laknas. We are still praying to do more and see where God can use us. Whenever we give to others, God blesses us right away in giving us a lot more in return.

I remember going to Marikaj for the first time to a youth camp organized by our church. Later on, I had come a couple of times as a visitor to the Tuesday night Bible lessons that are held there at the Hope Center for Teens by our pastor and with the help of a group from our church. Now that I am working for Hope for the World, I am here at the Hope Center in Marikaj daily as a part of God's great work here through Hope for the World.

Though I had a good job with the Film Company, during my last two years with them, I was really looking so forward to finding a new job. My family and my pastor were the only ones who knew how hungry I was to find a new job. The reason being that this job with the Film Company was taking *all of my time*. I had no time of my own any more. No time to serve the Lord. All my time and energy were spent on that job. Here in Albania, it is a luxury to have a good-paying job. And to look to move into another job would not be acceptable, so I had to keep it a secret and not tell anyone I was looking. I kept it as a prayer request just between me and God. All I did was pray and wait.

Right after I returned from my third trip to China for the Film Company, my pastor, Michael Fiocchi, told me that Perparim Demcellari of Hope for the World was looking for a lady to join their team. He asked me if I would want to have coffee with him and see if this opportunity would work well for both me and Hope for the World. A few days later, I had coffee with him. I had known Perparim for years as he was in my church and he and my first pastor were the ones who in 1994 came knocking on our door to invite us to the church.

I remembered that so well because my mom invited them inside. They came in and talked for hours. My grandparents were home that day, so Perparim and my grandpa, who had been in the military at the same time, did a lot of sharing of their stories from their military days. They also shared the gospel and asked my grandpa if he would mind if they would pray before they left. They prayed, even though my grandpa was raised in a family with very strong traditions as Muslims. In fact, his grandpa had spent his whole life as a Muslim priest.

That night, when my dad came home from work, my mom told him everything about the visitors and about the invitation to church. They both quickly agreed for my sister and I to go to the church because it would be a way for us to be around a better culture, and it was going to be a good opportunity to learn English. All of us Albanians love Americans and everything that has to do with them! Ha ha!

Right after their visit, my sister, Eni, and I started going to the church. Our grandma would help us to get there, and she would stay with us at the kids' program so she could tell my parents exactly what we did and what we heard, etc. After Eni and I started going to church, we began to invite lots of other kids from the neighborhood to join us because it was a very great experience. We had never seen or touched Muppets before, so doing this at church was something incredible.

We began to learn verses from the Bible, and were given candies. That was something. *Wow*! Singing songs with actions was something we had just seen in movies as growing up under communism in our country, the rule had been to stand stiff. That made you a great and model student. Since we had many friends coming with us to church, now my grandma didn't have to come with us.

I remember when my first pastor, David Young, and Perparim came again to our home for a visit, my mom asked Pastor David if we could play the piano sometimes in the church. He immediately agreed to start it little by little, and he loved the idea too. On that same day, they invited my grandparents to come to the church. It took some time for them to decide, but soon, since Eni and I had started to play in the church during offerings, or special dramas, etc., they started to come and followed us. They first started coming just for us, but later even if we were not doing something, they were still in the church. I remember when my grandpa first stepped his foot inside the church, everybody in our family, like cousins, etc., would react, "Wow! How did he make this decision, as he has been a strict Muslim all of his life?"

The truth is that my grandpa was a great man and really open-minded for that time. He had never forced my dad to go to the mosque. Although they said they were Muslim, they were not at all believers in that religion either. My grandpa had always been thirsty for knowledge, and he loved to read. He was brave during communism to even find books to read that were not allowed under the communist regime. He was open to hear as well, so I think this is the key that brought him to the church when he came.

Sorry, that took some time, now let's turn back to where I was when I had coffee with Perparim and he explained everything to me. He told me he would give me time to think about the job he was offering me with HFTW, but I told him, "I don't have anything to think about. This is all I have been praying for." So I started to work with HFTW on November 3, 2014.

Now, I'll share with you some of the best moments that I will never forget since I came to work with Hope for the World. When we first started a Kids Bible Club on Saturday mornings, the kids from the neighborhood would walk to our Hope Center. They were very aggressive and seemed to be interested only in causing problems. They were coming just to make a noise, joke with other kids, and make silly questions and would always throw stones when they would leave our grounds.

I remember one time we gave them some clothing for the beginning of the school year. Instead of carrying the clothing home, they threw them all in the pond near our property for no reason at all. They did this just because they had grown up with the mentality that "We are Muslim, and we do not need anything from Jesus." It was really very strange. They were doing all of these horrible things, but they were still faithfully coming every Saturday. In the beginning stages of our kids programs, all of our staff had to be ready to watch them as they came in because they were certainly thinking how they could cause some damage to our property.

The ones who had been the worst troublemakers were saved in the summer in our Vacation Bible School. The ones who would throw stones are the ones who now attend our teens program for ages fourteen and up on Tuesday nights. Many of them have been saved. They are participating in every program we have on different occasions. They are the ones helping us to share food boxes for the poor and elderly in the community at Christmas. They also are the ones going with us door-to-door singing the Christmas carols. They help us always in different activities, sharing invitations, keeping the crowd of kids in line, setting up chairs, and cleaning up after an event. This really has proven to me that "All things work together for good to those who love the Lord" as it says in Romans 8:28.

The kids program began on March 14, 2014, and continues every week to this day. The only problem we have with troublemakers now is they want to win every game, get nervous really quick playing, arguing with each other, ha ha ha. That's part of every Albanian's makeup, a very competitive spirit. There's nothing wrong with them, and they have become great now and participate well in all activities.

I grew up in church with struggles, because it was the first church we had after cCommunism fell. But struggles in Marikaj have been even bigger. Because it's not in the city and people are not as open-minded as the ones who have lived or grown up in the capital city of Tirana. You may have parents here that agree that their daughter can come and attend the service we have for the teens only if you come and pick her up at home, by walking *not* by car. If you go by car, they will not allow you to take her because they are afraid what neighbors may think that their daughter went somewhere in a car. They don't mind that you have to walk twenty to thirty minutes instead of going with a car. And if you tell them you will bring their daughter back in one hour, it had better be just one hour. If not, you'll be in trouble. Parents here in Marikaj will allow their daughters to come to church when the days get longer, and it's not dark but not if it's wintertime, and 4:00 p.m. sounds pretty late to them. On Saturday mornings, you can't have a meeting for the young ladies, because they all are cleaning at their homes. It's the same rules in every home. They are part of a mentality that is keeping them away from so many good things. We are praying for some special times with the young girls and young ladies of the village.

Working in the orphanage has been one of my sweetest responsibilities, too. I grew up in a family where if we desired to have a new doll, or new book, sometimes parents would provide it, sometimes they would explain to us why they can't afford it for us. But I truly matured in the Lord when I would see kids in the orphanage saying prayers "for mom to get out from the jail as soon as she can" or pray "that my dad will take me from here if he gets out of jail, so we can live together" or pray for a whole year that "I can have a pair of tennis shoes" or "I pray I can have more than one dress when I get older," because she has just one dress. One beautiful dress per child would be kept by workers at the orphanage for each child as a treasure to use it just for special events. The rest of the year, the girls would be dressed like a boy. And sometimes their hair would be cut (shaved in the summer time) so they never really had a chance to look pretty like a girl.

I recall one special prayer by Demokrat Lloci. "I pray for my younger sister after she leaves the orphanage to be able to go to the Hope Center. I don't care for myself. I'm a boy, and I'll find a way to make it, I want so hard for her to have a real home." This prayer was answered, by the way, and his sister is now at the Hope Center.

This may sound crude, but I have really experienced these things while working with orphan children. I have seen that most of them, not all, at the orphanage tend to be very unthankful and lazy. They take things for granted, they expect a lot from others, but they hardly think to help themselves by thinking or doing something. This has always burdened me about the orphans. We try very hard at the Hope Center for Teens to reverse that kind of thinking and attitude. One day in Korca at the baby orphanage, we took two of the teens who are a part of the Hope Center. When we finished the Muppet program with our teenage girls, they were so touched seeing those little precious babies. They couldn't hold the tears for hours, saying, "We have been just like these babies. They don't know their biological families, but Hope for the World will be like their own family for years." From that day forward, a lot of things in the lives of these two young ladies has changed, and their attitudes have changed greatly. They became humble and live now with the desire of what they can do for others, how they can help, and how they can be involved in God's work. This is one of the greatest missions of Hope for the World, changing the lives of orphans and helping them become servants of the Lord.

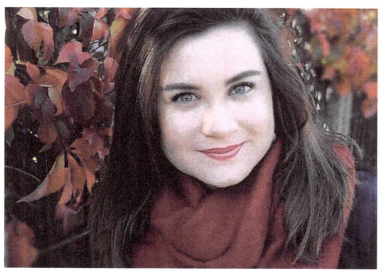

Ledina Rabdishta
Such a wonderful staff member.
Administrative Assistant at the Hope Center
Secretary to President Perparim Demcellari

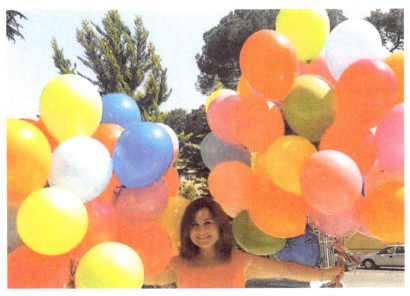

Ledina and Balloons for orphan's day at the Zyber
Halluli Orphanage in Tirana. She always has
Something very exciting for them on these days I

Our Work in Saranda

Before I share the testimonies of Fatos and Mirela Demiri, our staff team working in Saranda, Albania, I want to say that we had been ministering to orphans for many years and Roger always claimed James 1:27 as the verse on which he felt called to work in Albania. This verse says:

> *Pure and undefiled religion before God and the Father is this: to visit orphans and widows in their trouble, and to keep oneself unspotted from the world.*

One day, I went to Roger, and I said, "You know what, honey? We aren't really fulfilling that whole verse in James because we are not helping take care of the widows in Albania."

He says in jest that he really wanted to smack me one when I brought that up as he knew it meant we'd have to add more funds to our already heavy budget. But sure enough, it wasn't too long after that when we were asked by Fatos in Saranda if we would be able to start helping the elderly center in Saranda where widows, and also widowers, gathered every day to spend time together. They had many needs at the center, for repairs, and things like a nice kitchen in which to prepare meals for the elderly each day. They needed all of the things to supply the kitchen, appliances, cookware, dishes, and silverware. Actually, the entire kitchen needed to be remodeled and supplied in order to make this elderly center efficient for the group of fifty or sixty precious senior citizens.

There was no problem at all in us bringing them Bibles and speakers and teachers and missionaries who were in the area to tell them about Jesus. After all, they were actually at the crucial stage when they needed to come to know Christ as life on earth for them was getting shorter daily. So we began with a regular monthly budget to help them with their needs at the center and also brought in groups from America to do work projects at this center, which we called the Threshold of Hope. They have actually moved to another location in recent years, and it is much better suited for their needs. However, there are still many things to be done even at this new location. We plan to work on these projects as soon as possible.

One of the key friends and project coordinators we have had working in Saranda through our years in Albania has been Chris Martin, from our same hometown, McDonough, Georgia. He was first with a church in the area that would send groups of men and women to Saranda on many, many occasions to assist Chris in the maintenance projects both at the Threshold of Hope as well as at the school-age orphanage there in Saranda that housed a large number of children.

We asked Chris recently how many people he had taken over there to work through the years, and he said it was about seventy that he could remember and count. He has made about fifteen different trips to do work and not only to do work physically but to be a blessing to the children and to the workers there. He and his wife, Sandy, actually adopted one of the girls from the orphanage there after a few visits. And other friends from his group and church adopted siblings, two girls, into their family. There were other adoptions by more people who had come over there with Chris and fallen in love with these kids. There's really just no telling what the overall influence has been on this Saranda ministry through the love and caring of this brother.

We are happy to have Chris as a member of our church now. He is getting together his second work and ministry team from Glen Haven Baptist. They will make a trip shortly to continue doing some projects that are badly needed. He and his wife and their business have also been a blessing financially to help us keep the work going with the Threshold of Hope seniors. We thank God for giving him a heart for this work years ago, and he has remained faithful to help continually; even when he could not go at times, he would always help us financially.

I wanted you to know a little bit about the beginnings of our work with the widows, but now I am going to introduce you to Fatos and Mirela Demiri and their family who have played an immense role in our ministry in Albania from the very beginning when Hope for the World went there originally to plant the first evangelical church in Saranda, Albania, after communism fell.

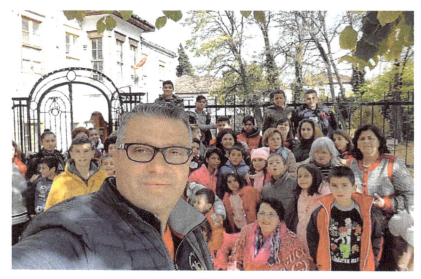

Fatos' Testimony
Photo Is Fatos with the kids from Saranda Orphanage
On a very special trip to the City of Korea.

THE MAKING OF A WONDERFUL LIFE

Fatos's Testimony

I started working for Hope for the World in 2002. In September 2002, I met the director of HFTW Albania, Roger Mullins, and he talked with me about their work with the orphans. At the beginning, I worked together with an American missionary, Mike Bebout, and when he left Albania, I started to do the work at the orphanage by myself for Hope for the World. It was such a hard time for the children there, and they were kids with different stories and problems. But the worst thing I saw was that nobody was there to speak to them about God. In the beginning of democracy in Albania, after the fall of communism, in the year 1993, in Saranda, there came a lot of American missionaries in the name of Hope for the World. At the same time, they created the first Baptist church in Saranda. I started to go to the church, and in July 1995, I was saved and baptized. A lot of bad things happened in my life. The worst thing was the accidental premature death of the most important person for me, my father. But even through this hard trial in my life, I never lost faith in God. So it was easy for me to speak to these kids about God and his job and plans for their lives. During all these years, these kids have been growing together with us and in God's Word, and I am so happy that HFTW is present in Saranda, as such a spiritual help as well as a material one.

Editor's note: Fatos takes a very personal interest in each one of the kids at the orphanage. When he sees that they are gifted in some special area of art, or music, for instance, he has provided much help personally and then found others, including our organization, to contribute to the needs for special tutoring, art classes and music lessons. He has made sure that there have been instruments like keyboards, violins, and guitars purchased and teachers provided to give lessons to the kids who have these talents. Then he encourages them to use their talents in the church and in special programs around the town. It has been amazing to see how God has been helping these kids find some wonderful self-worth by learning to do these things and taking pride in using their gifts. Something else about Fatos, that he is too humble to tell you, is that he and his mother, Hene, who was widowed very young, together with Fatos's younger brother, Mendi, have been operating a beautiful guesthouse which they started with just one floor, then added another, and another, and yet another and now have a beautiful structure where we all stay when we go to Saranda. It is a profitable business for the family, and they serve a wonderful home-cooked breakfast under the grape arbor on their patio every morning. Hene does most of the work connected with the guesthouse now, because both of her boys are married with children and doing other jobs away from the home. However, it is not uncommon to have Fatos and Mendi serving up breakfast to us mornings when we visit. It's a great family guesthouse, and we have spent many, many wonderful hours of Christian fellowship with brothers and sisters in Christ whom we have brought from America to visit the work in Albania. Saranda also is a place of ancient biblical historical sites. The town of Butrinti is there, and you can see the ruins of early Christian churches and amphitheaters that were built in the days of Apostle Paul. It is noted in the Bible that he visited this country. Look in your Bible maps and in the scriptures for "Illyrica." That is ancient Albania. It is so worth a stop in Saranda if for no other reason than to see these wonderful archeological digs from biblical days. Saranda is always our last stop on our tour of the orphanages, as it is the farthest point south in the country, and we take a ferry across to Greece and tour the beautiful Greek island of Corfu before we leave to return home to America.

And now, a word from Mirela, the sweet wife of Fatos.

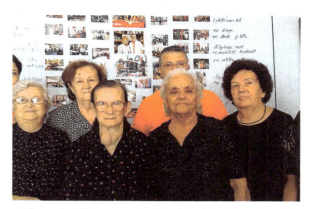

Photo is of Fatos and wife, Mirela with a few of
The widows we minister to each month.

THE MAKING OF A WONDERFUL LIFE

Mirela's Testimony

My first contact with HFTW was when the wonderful couple, Roger and Cherie Mullins, blessed our marriage in September 2004. My husband had been working for HFTW since 2002, and he had talked so many times about his job in the first years we got to know each other. Staying together with all the people who came in our guesthouse in Saranda and listening to their testimonies, I realized that these people were connected to each other by a very special power that was the power of God.

During these early years of our marriage, I was a bank employee, and I was working so very hard at my job, even extra hours. It took me away from my family so much. It was a winter evening in 2009 when I had a phone call from Bro. Roger Mullins, and he asked me to work as a part-time worker for HFTW. I accepted, of course. I have been privileged to work with the kids at the orphanage ever since then. I also go to the Threshold of Hope and love on the widows and help Fatos in any activities he plans for them. The first time I met the kids at the orphanage, and when they all ran toward me to hug me, I felt like the happiest person in the world. Being already the mother of two boys, and having myself grown up as a child without a father, I could realize better than anyone the need of these kids for affection and love. There, I realized that even if we are well dressed or not, well educated or not, rich or poor, it doesn't matter. Before God, we are all equal. So HFTW and the people involved with them changed my life and the lives of these children. Thank you, God, for directing our lives. We feel so safe with you.

Editor's note: Mirela is a very sweet friend to me, and she and I have spent some very special times talking together about the things of God and about parenting and marriage. I have enjoyed having them in our home in Georgia on different occasions. Their two boys are growing up now and are beginning to help their dad in the family business of tourism that is flourishing in Saranda. If you ever want to visit Saranda, you can't go wrong by selecting Terini Travel in Saranda to handle your trip for you.

Fatos coordinates tours in all of Albania, Greece, Macedonia, and other areas around Albania, as well. This country is one of the best-kept secrets in all of Europe, but it is getting better known every year. Many tourists from European countries love to go there, and some are buying condos to rent out to tourists. Hotels are being built along the seacoast, creating a beautiful Albanian Riviera along the Adriatic and Ionian Seas. People have asked us what it is like to go on a tour of the orphanages with us. We have taken many, many people with us to Albania through the years. Well, it's more like a lovely vacation with orphan kids thrown in to make you laugh or cry. You can feel free to hug them, and they will want to entertain you. And they will definitely grab your heart. We are always accompanied by our Albanian Christian staff. We have our own drivers who are employed by HFTW. They are very capable drivers and will take great care of us wherever we go in Albania. In fact, we will travel in a nice new VW van that we have purchased in recent years. We stay in good hotels, with private baths in each room. Rooms are very, very clean. They are also air-conditioned. The food is excellent in the restaurants. We always feel like family as we travel together for those ten days in Albania. The spirit of the trip is awesome. The beauty of the country is breathtaking. You are much safer in Albania than you are on any city street in America. We are always in a group. Our day is full of activity from morning until night. There is very little "free time," but we do try to arrange some time for shopping at some point in the trip. There will be a few touristic things we will do while in the country as there are some very beautiful sites and ancient ruins, castles, etc., to visit.

Albanians love America, and they love American people!

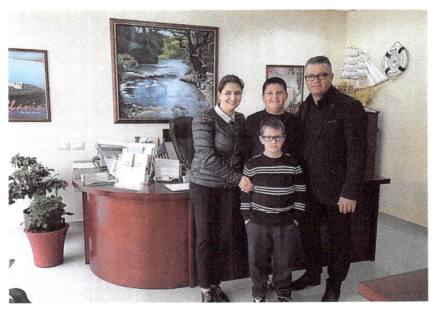

Here's a photo of the Demiri Family...
Mirela, Fatos, Ani and Rei
They all work hard in our ministry as well As
their own Tourism Business in Saranda.

Buddy's Thoughts

I remember the first time that I went to Albania, my parents had been working with the orphans for seven years. I was utterly amazed at how extensive the work was, how many lives were being reached, the beauty of the country, and yet the desperate need they had. I recall attending a couple of government meetings with my father and being overwhelmed at the favor God had given him with these leaders of the country. There were so many open doors to Hope for the World from those who were making decisions for the entire country of Albania, not only the orphanages. Everywhere we would go, and in whatever meeting we would be involved, the national leaders and government directors of the orphanages would share their desire to have Hope for the world involved. I noticed that many times, they wanted Hope for the World to lead the way and help them lay plans for future programs for the orphans of Albania. We have to say that much of this was because of the tremendous staff led by Hope for the World's in-country president, Perparim Demcellari. They have all worked together as a well-oiled machine to keep the reputation of Hope for the World in Albania spotless. They have even been listed as the leading nongovernmental organization (NGO) in Albania. They have held to their word and seen to it that every contract they have entered into throughout the years has been honored and fulfilled.

Something else that truly made a huge impression on me was in the last year that George W. Bush was president of the United States, he and Mrs. Laura Bush made a trip to Albania. He was the very first president of the United States who had ever visited

Albania. Mrs. Bush had sent a team into Albania ahead of their visit to seek out some American organizations who were truly making an impact on the Albanian society. They spent some time with government officials asking about any American NGOs that were truly making a difference in their country. They reported to them that Hope for the World was one and another was Bethany Adoption Services. She determined that when she would be coming to Albania, she wanted to meet with leaders and some of the teenagers who were being helped in the teen center by Hope for the World. The day arrived, and the meetings for both groups were held at the location of Bethany's baby orphanage in Tirana, Albania. Hope for the World's president, Perparim Demcellari, and other staff workers and teens from Hope for the World got to meet with Mrs. Bush personally. She interviewed some of the teens who were living in HFTW's teen center at that time. She was very impressed with these young people and they with her. It was a very memorable occasion for HFTW, and they felt so blessed to have this visit from the first lady of America. I remember hearing that when Mrs. Bush asked one of the young ladies if she had any questions for her, she replied, "Yes, Mrs. Bush, are you a Christian?" Mrs. Bush smiled and did not hesitate to respond very quickly that she certainly was a Christian and she was so happy she had asked her that question.

On a more personal note, Kerri and I had been sponsoring a child for a few years. His name was Ergys. I was really looking forward to meeting him when we arrived in Shkoder and went to the school-age orphanage there. I can still remember how they led me to an office where Ergys and one of our interpreters were waiting for me. The moment we saw each other, it was as if we were family. Ergys hugged me so tight and just held on to me for so long that sweat began to pour off of us both. He did not want to let go. Finally, after some time, we shared some light conversation as I gave him a gift and some things Victoria and Olivia (our girls) had sent over to him like pictures they had drawn of our family where they included Ergys with us. I mean, it was a very emotional time together, one I will never forget. A few minutes later, they had it prepared for me to sing a few songs for the kids in a recreation room with a stage. Really, all I can say about that is it's a miracle that I even made it through the songs. One song that I had written back then was entitled "Child of the Father," and the chorus says:

> You're a child of the Father
> You mean everything to me
> You've already been accepted
> Just crawl up here on my knee
> I'll wrap my arms around you
> I'll whisper to your soul
> You're a child of the Father
> And I'll never let you go

As I got to that chorus, I sat down on the edge of the stage, and here came Ergys and a few other kids crawling up there around me as I pulled them up next to me, weeping, because I had never had words of any song mean more to me than these did at that moment.

Over these past fifteen years, I have made many more trips to Albania, as well as my wife, Kerri, and both of our daughters, Victoria and Olivia. Hope for the World Albania has changed our lives as a family. In 2013, Kerri and I surrendered to work with Hope for the World which has now grown from the work in Albania into works in Romania, India, Ukraine, Honduras, and Ethiopia. In 2015, we stepped out full-time to represent these amazing fields of service and those who sacrifice to love the "least of these." It is such a great honor to be a part of this life-changing work.

In June of 2017, I had the privilege to accompany my dad, Roger Mullins, and Jimmy and Janice Franks, the founders of Hope For The World, together with a couple of other pastors, as we went to Albania for the celebration of twenty-five years of Hope for the World working with children in the orphanages of Albania. The HFTW staff in Albania had put together an amazing event that was held in the courtyard of the Sheraton Hotel in Tirana. There were so many things about this night that were a blessing to me, but I believe what stood out to me the most was that over half of those in attendance were from the Albanian government and social services. One of the special guest speakers was then the director of social services, I believe her name was Etleva Bisha. She was a brilliant speaker. One of the most memorable statements she made in her speech was that Hope for the World had not simply changed the lives of the children in the orphanages in Albania but that it had changed the country of Albania.

The speakers for the evening consisted of Jimmy Franks, speaking about the beginning of Hope for the World in Albania back in 1992. My dad, Roger Mullins, who spoke of the wonderful relationship he had experienced working in Albania these twenty-five years as the director of operations from the US offices. He also presented some special recognition plaques to HFTW President Perparim Demcellari and special certificates to each of the directors of the orphanages with whom we have been involved in Albania. Another occasion that was recognized was the retirement of one of the men on the Shkoder staff, Mr. Nikolin Lekaj, who had worked with HFTW for eighteen years.

Most big events build up to a high-powered, big-named, popular speaker to close the night out, but what was truly moving to me was that the keynote speaker for this night was one of the young ladies named Manuela, who had come through the orphanages and the Hope Center for Teens. She had graduated from high school the year before and was now in college preparing for her own career and future. Another of the young ladies who offered the official greeting for the night had also grown up in the Tirana orphanage and then moved to Hope for the World's Hope Center for Teens. Her name was Mbresa. Her older sister and younger brother had also come through the Hope Center and graduated from high school. She was a big part of the evening and in keeping the program running smoothly. She was an excellent student and was making a great contribution to their society in her country. This was truly unheard of for orphans years ago in Albania and is a living testimony of what God's love can do when we put it in action. To see hope like that displayed gives thousands of others who felt they had no hope, the desire to overcome. Hope for the World is Christ's love manifested through us so that others may know they truly have a hope for the future.

I am so blessed to be a part of this great work that God began in Albania in 1992 and that I am sure will continue growing in Albania. I am so glad to see that the work of Hope for the World has been so designed that as long as the necessary funds are provided, it can continue to thrive for future generations. The leadership is all in place within the country, and the nationals are doing an awesome job in every location. I do appreciate so much the work of my parents in putting together a wonderful staff in Albania to carry out this tremendous ministry. Only God knows what is on the horizon for Hope for the World Albania.

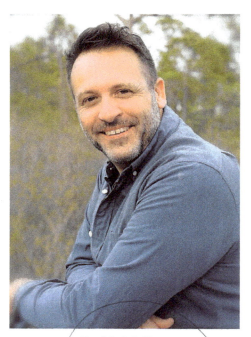

Buddy Mullins
CEO of Hope for the World Foundation

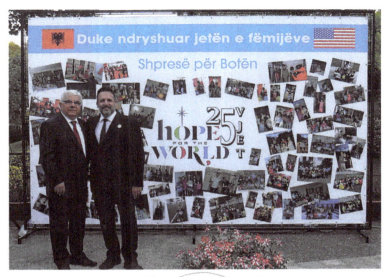

Pictured here are Buddy with our
In-Country President—Perparim Demcellari At
the 25th Celebration of HFTW in Albania

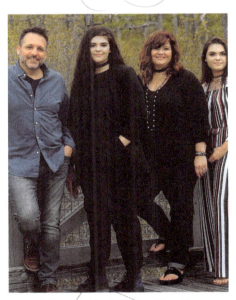

The Buddy Mullins Family
Buddy, Olivia, Kerri and Victoria
All of them have been to Albania several times.

Kerri Says

After a grueling forty-eight-hour trip in airplanes and extended layovers in airports because of flight overbooking in Europe, we finally arrived in the middle of the night at Tirana, Albania, and the Mother Theresa airport. (A bit of trivia here: it is named for Mother Theresa as she was born and raised in Shkoder, Albania. We have walked down the street where she was born many times while visiting there.) We then took a very bumpy ride in a van for about three hours and finally made it to our hotel in Shkoder to sleep.

The next day, we were greeted by Fredi and Prenda and their new baby, Edona. We visited the baby orphanage first and loved on the toddlers and held the babies in our arms, hearing the stories of how this one was dropped off in a basket on the front stoop or that one was illegitimate and the mom couldn't afford to keep it. It broke my heart to think of a baby, so sweet and beautiful, not being loved in the arms of its own mom or dad. However, seeing the love shown by Prenda, our HFTW staff member, and the other workers was a blessing. They were kissing each one and calling them by their names, and the toddlers would run, holding their arms up to be held. I just knew God was taking care of these little ones.

What would seemingly be the worst thing that could happen to a child, to be without a mom or dad who cared for them, God completely turned around. He truly left none of them out of his care, and he sent Roger and Cherie and Hope for the World to care for these babies and all the other children in the many orphanages throughout the twenty-five years Hope for the World has been in Albania. It is a blessing knowing that many babies have been adopted into Christian homes from these orphanages through the years.

We then drove to the school-age orphanage, and I got to meet my little guy we had been sponsoring since he was two years old. His name was Ergys, pronounced like "Air Goose." I remember looking at pictures of children from this orphanage and picking him out because of his amazing smile. Here was this dark-skinned black-haired tiny boy with the prettiest white-toothed grin I had ever seen. I just knew he was the one we were to help. Well, when we got out of the van and I saw him for the first time, he ran up to me and gave me a huge hug with that same big white-toothed grin on his beautiful face. He clung to me the entire time we were there. I gave him some gifts from us, he showed us his room, and then we were able to spend some time talking with him through an interpreter. I told him through tears that my greatest desire for him was that he come to know Jesus and ask him into his heart. He shook his head, and I know that later in his life, he did exactly that.

Ergys is now a grown man and has gone back to live and work with his uncle in a town not too many miles from the city of Shkoder where I met him. I hear from our staff workers that he is doing just fine, and that blesses us. There is a church in his town, and he is a part of that church.

Later on, we visited the Tag Center for Teens in Tirana, the capital city, and although we had refurbished it through the funds raised by our friend, Fred Tag, who you read about in this book, and they had nice things in the facility, it was a building owned by the Albanian government, and they were taking back more and more of it for government offices. It was making the Tag Center too small to care for more than six or eight kids. I remember thinking we needed a new facility to house more teens and came back with a burden to see that happen, I wasn't the only one with that burden, and you have read how God allowed us to have our very own property in Marikaj, Albania. It is a good two and a half acre piece of property with two buildings that are just what we needed. So we now have the Hope Center for Teens, where we are equipped to house so many more and are more able to minister to these kids and prepare them for a future full of hope.

I have been amazed to see what God could do through ordinary people who sacrifice their time, their money, and their talents to help these young orphan children in Albania. It takes everyone working together on both sides of the water. It would not have been possible without the wonderful sponsors and donors who keep the funds provided month after month and year after year.

Buddy and I are so blessed to be a part of God's family working with our brothers and sisters in Christ who live with these orphan children and provide love they had never received. We are all like one big family when we get to visit over there. This love is truly one that will stay with them throughout their lives as it is the love of our Savior, and it is everlasting. Temporary homes, whether in Albanian orphanages or in American family dwellings, are nothing compared to the eternal home we will share with them in heaven one day.

Editor's note: We are so blessed to have Kerri as our daughter-in-law. She has been the perfect helpmeet for our son all of the years they have been married, since 1990. She works with Buddy side by side in their ministry for the Hope for the World Foundation in Santa Rosa Beach, Florida. They are involved daily in encouraging all of us who are doing mission work under Hope for the World. They keep newsletters going out, social media updated, and personal words of encouragement as well as financial aid coming to each of the directors on the fields of Albania, Ethiopia, Honduras, India, Romania, and Ukraine. They have made visits to most all of these countries and will complete their coverage by visiting the remaining one very shortly. They stay busy during the year presenting Hope for the World Foundation's work to churches and many other gatherings of people in America. They are continually raising awareness for each of us in the various countries.

Kerri and I have a similar calling and service in life, that is, working with our husbands twenty-four hours a day, seven days a week. That is something that is not easy at times but is always rewarding. We thank God for Kerri. She is a blessing in our lives and comes from a very wonderful family, Tom and Merleene King, of Gadsden, Alabama. They raised her to serve the Lord, and she has not disappointed them. Kerri graduated from Liberty University where she was a music major. That has also worked in such a special way into their music ministry as a family. Their daughters, Victoria and Olivia, make up the rest of their family, and I'm proud and happy to say that all of them are loving God and serving him with their talent. We love Kerri so much and thank God for putting her in our family.

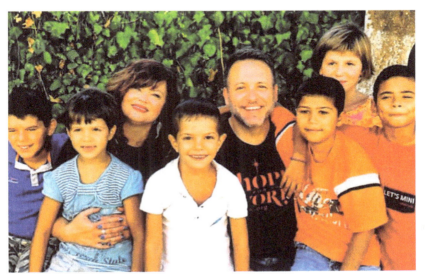

Kerri and Buddy with a group of children
From the Saranda Orphanage—2018.

Roger's Reflections

You know, since Cherie has been writing this book for the past two or three years, she and I have spent some very special times just reflecting on the blessings that have been ours to share in this particular phase of our various ministries we have had since our marriage in 1962. We actually sit in restaurants many times and just go over the many places we have lived since we were married, and I believe that number is sixteen, but if I add in the three buses we lived in while in evangelism, that would be nineteen different places in fifty-seven years. That averages out to nearly a move every three years, but the moving was mostly done before 1996, because since then, we have lived here in this house in McDonough, Georgia. We've been here twenty-three years as of 2019, the year we are trying to get this book of Cherie's published! So in our young years, you might say we were a'hustlin' about from pillar to post so to speak. I'm an old Tennessee boy, so you have to forgive the way I might slaughter the King's English.

Cherie would have it no other way than for me to think up a couple of the stories in Albania that she hadn't already thought of for me and written about so very "purty" in this here book, so I've been a'thinkin' and a'thinkin' these past few days, and I came up with a couple that just might interest some of you who are readin' my writin'.

One of the very first missionaries into Albania was a man, David Young, and his wife, Faye. They were great people, but they were from the north. Now I ain't got nothin' against northerners, because you see, I married a Yankee girl, but I got her out of there as quick as I could. You might say I rescued her! Well, David and I could fellowship all day long about the things of God, the Bible, bringing people to Christ, missions, Albanian folks, and all sorts of wonderful topics, but we really had quite a difference of opinion when it came to Christian music. You see, he came up in the churches that expected every singer to stand stiff as a board behind the pulpit and just sing—straight voiced—and without any physical moving and without much vocal movement either. I think he might really like the educated vocalists rather than us good old down-home country southern gospel harmonizers. But he was kind enough to allow me to sing in his church from time to time. One or two of my songs may have been all right for him. I heard that the people really enjoyed my singin', and that's why he would ask me to sing when I would come over there. I used to tease David big time about our music differences. In fact, once my wife jokingly sent him some tapes, she found somewhere that were recorded as "funeral music." She thought he might enjoy them or at least get a good laugh.

Well, one particular time, when I was in Albania, Brother David was going way up into the mountains to minister in a village area where they had thought about starting a church, if they could get a group of folks saved up there. He told me he would love to take me up there to sing outside on the road right at a place where there was a community bar. He had come to know the bar owner pretty well (don't ask me how), and he said it was OK with him if we came right there on his property and sang and preached and tried to gather up a crowd. I guess he thought if we brought them in, then he'd get him some customers.

We rode up there in David's Land Rover, and I happened to have soundtracks with me that I sang with. Then David told me they didn't have any electricity up there, and I said, "Well, how in the world am I gonna sing with no way to play my tape player and soundtracks?"

David assured me it would be OK and not to worry about it. Well, sure enough! We got there after a long, long climb up steep mountains that had no guardrails on the edge of the roads, and the roads were all dirt and rocks and very, very treacherous. I will say this,

I was prayed up by the time I got there as I'd been in touch with God the entire ride.

David lifted up the hood of the Land Rover, and he hooked some wires in a way that we could connect my tape player and play those tapes as long as the engine kept running, and we didn't run out of gas. It's a blessing that I was born with a good set of lungs, I guess, as I had to be able to sing over the hum of the engine while breathing in the exhaust fumes. Of course, I had been used to diesel fumes, having lived on a bus for years in our evangelism days.

I had some really peppy tunes I could sing, and it began to bring out the children first. Here they came, gathering around to hear me sing. Brother David and some others he had with him were equipped with some gospel tracts in the Albanian language to give out to the people who showed up and of course he was a wonderful one-on-one personal soul winner, but he had to have his interpreter right beside him the whole time. Soon some adults gathered around, too, and the owner of the bar came out to meet me and to welcome us and told us to stay as long as we wanted.

It was an awesome experience, and I believe some seeds were truly planted on that occasion because they did start a church there, right in that bar! They let them have a back room to meet with the people, and we went back there again from time to time. I even took my pastor, Ralph Easterwood, up there with us once, and he was amazed at this place and the extreme poverty we saw in the village surrounding this bar.

Well, the main thing I wanted to tell you was that while we were there, a very old gentleman came over to me and spoke to me through my interpreter saying that he wanted me to please come down to his house, he had something very important he wanted to show me. Well, now, we were way, way up a mountain. I asked him where he lived, and he pointed way down a little path down the mountain. Now I will have to admit that I am a man of pride, and way too much at times, and I had on a brand spankin' new pair of blue jeans that day. Also, it had rained some before we got there that day, and that path looked mighty slick and slimy. I could just imagine tryin' to maneuver that slippery path down that steep hill to that old man's house, and I nearly refused, but the Lord wouldn't let me. He seemed like a very sweet man and I could see a special glow on his face and light in his eye.

So off we went. He led the way, of course, I was second, and like I said, I nearly slid down that hill like a slide on my rear end the whole way. My interpreter was behind me laughing out loud. My poor white tennis shoes were all muddy, and my new jeans were wet and muddy, but we finally arrived at our destination, a little hut there at the foot of the hill. It had a dirt floor in it, but he had a nicely swept carpet over the dirt floor. He invited me inside, and then he proceeded to show me a hole he had in one of the walls. It was about eighteen inches in diameter, sort of a circle. Then he told me the story of why that hole was there.

He said, "In 1947, when communism took over this country, they took all of our Bibles away from us and burned them all in the middle of the villages." He said, "I loved my Bible, and I loved the Lord, and I didn't want them burning my Bible, so I punched a hole in my wall here, and I hid my Bible down inside the wall, and I had to leave it there until 1992 when the communist wall finally fell. I was just a young man when I hid my Bible, but now I'm an old man, but I was so happy for the day I could bust a hole in that wall and get out my Bible."

He went over to the table and picked it up and held it in his arms like a baby, and he kissed it and kissed it and hugged it tight to his chest. My heart exploded inside of me at that moment because I thought, *Oh my goodness, Roger, do you love your Bible like this old man loves his?* I truly got convicted right there in that old man's home that day. I never ever forgot that experience or that day, and I go back in my thought closet and pull that dear memory out every once in a while and ask God to give me the love I need to have, and like that old man had, for God's Word. I thank God for allowing me to get my blue jeans dirty for such a wonderful lesson that has stuck with me for more than twenty years now. Praise the Lord!

There's another time that God was truly looking out for me on one of my very first trips to Albania. I had taken one of my dearest friends, Roger Ver Lee, from Grand Rapids, Michigan, with me.

Roger had been very, very helpful to me for years during our evangelism days. He was used by the Lord to help us get our second bus back then. We also went on some other mission trips together to Belize, South America, when I was in evangelism. Well, it was only natural for me to ask him to go with me to Albania when I began working in that country, and it was more than natural for him to say yes and to come. He had a heart as big as all outdoors when it came to helping people. I cannot think of a time when I needed help in some way that Roger wasn't there to help. He was a great blessing in Albania as well. I remember walking him through one of the orphanages where the little kids were in bed taking naps in the middle of the day. It was wintertime. There was no heat in the orphanage, and they were tucked in tightly with wool blankets on their tiny metal cots. It was so cold that you could see the breath of each child as they slept. Well, that got such a hold on Roger that he asked me right then and there to see what we could do about putting some heat in that orphanage. So we discussed this need with the director and found out what it would cost to put in a new diesel-burning furnace to heat the place. It was costly, but Roger promised to send the funds right back as soon as he got home, and this he did. He was a man of his word.

Well, that was a little side story, and praise to the Lord for providing heat in that big orphanage in Shkoder that we had just taken on by faith a little before this trip. Back to my original planned story now.

Roger and I had been invited by David Young to go with him to another village that was a long drive away and up in the mountains again, the village of Berat, I believe it was. We were going there to meet a family that he was witnessing to. So off we went again in the Land Rover. We got there, and we were welcomed into this home up there, and the people were very, very poor, but, oh, so friendly to us and so happy to have Americans visiting them.

They sat us all around a big table, and we just sat there and drank Turkish coffee and talked, and David shared the Word of God with them, and we had a wonderful time, but we had to leave so we could get back home before too late as the next day was Sunday as

I recall. Well, when we got all the way back to Tirana that night, I realized that I had lost my passport, and I believed I had left it there at that house way up there six hours away. Oh, my goodness! What was I to do? There was no way to call them and ask about it, but our wonderful driver who had driven us up and back that whole trip that day turned right around and went back that long way just to see if my passport was there. It was a scary thing to lose your passport in Albania as they could sell an American passport to some mafia people for $10,000. I just knew that my passport would be for sale, and I would never see it again. Well, I'm telling you the truth. That driver got up there, and I saw him early the next morning down at the restaurant underneath the rooms where we were staying at the Stephen Center, and he was waving my passport. They had found it, and they were protecting it for me. It was safe and sound, and I was so relieved and so blessed at the same time to know that these were such good people. I began at that time to truly love and trust these Albanian people. God was truly knitting our hearts together and making a very strong *Albanian Attachment.*

Just before I write the Epilogue, I want to add a special chapter or two that I feel led of the Lord to share. It will lead nicely into the Epilogue, and you'll see why. Thank you so much for reading my final book in my series entitled *The Making of a Wonderful Life.* If you haven't read the three preceding this, they are subtitled *Recording Reflections, Family Foundations, and Joyous Journey.*

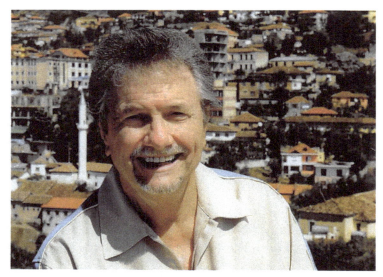

One of my favorite pictures of Roger in Albania.
Ancient City of Kruja in the background.

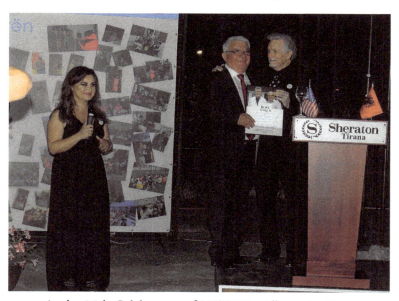

At the 25th Celebration of HFTW in Albania in 2017
Roger presents a special plaque Perparim Demcellari.
He has been our Albanian President of HFTW since 1999.
He has been a God-send to us throughout the years.

Roger's Double Whammy

It was in the year *2015* that Roger had two very serious physical attacks. I remember like it was yesterday that Monday morning, the day after Mother's Day. Roger turned on the TV in the bedroom when he got up and began to get frantic because there was a loud static noise. He called me in there and said, "Cherie, what's wrong with our TV?" I guess he thought maybe I had done something to it, I don't know. I told him that I didn't understand what he meant because to me it sounded perfectly normal. He said that all he could hear was roaring distortion and static. He could not understand anything. He then went out to the living room and checked that TV. It was the same there. He began to get very anxious and upset. His ears were going crazy, and he was hearing all kinds of roars and sounds he had never heard before.

I immediately made an appointment with his ENT to see if they could help him. They just diagnosed it as tinnitus and said there's not really a cure for that. It is something that only the patient can hear inside of his head, and there is no remedy that they knew of. They did all the normal testing to his ears and also checked his "high-dollar" hearing aids he had bought within the last two or three years. They were working correctly. Nothing seemed to relieve this noise he was experiencing. It was nearly driving him crazy and making him have much anxiety. The anxiety made him lose his appetite, and he began to lose weight almost daily. Every doctor visit he would have after that, he would have lost a few more pounds.

We searched the Internet, reading all kinds of things about tinnitus. We even downloaded a book on the subject, and it was there that we read that all sorts of medications could cause this type of side effect. Roger even made a decision to quit taking one in particular without consulting with his physician.

He just began to try different things to help relieve the ringing. I know when it would be its worst, he would just go outside and run around the block because they did say that exercise would improve it, and he had not been one to do a lot of physical exercise, outside of playing golf occasionally. Living with tinnitus. Many people have that and have to manage it in their lives. Roger was now one of those and was trying to reach some type of normal. This event also caused him more hearing loss in both ears. His left ear has a very low percentage of hearing and thus makes it impossible for him to sing any more. That was one of the things he loved most to do in his service for the Lord, and it was now gone completely. We would love to insert a praise, however, that as he was a veteran of the USAF, a friend of ours insisted that he go to the Veterans Administration in Decatur, Georgia, and let them test his ears and fit him with the very best state-of-the-art hearing aids. This we did in January of 2017, and they have made a tremendous improvement for him with his tinnitus problem. He seldom complains of having that roaring noise any more.

The second whammy hit him the last day of October 2015 when he was visiting a friend in the hospital who had recently had a massive stroke. His friend, Jeff, was paralyzed, couldn't talk, and was in rough shape after his stroke. While Roger was standing there praying over Jeff, all of a sudden, he noticed his own words becoming indistinguishable even to himself. He seemed to be babbling and mumbling and could not even make out what he was trying to say in his prayer. It shook him up so much that he just left quickly, got in his car, and drove home.

How I have wished that I had been with him to hear that. I would have known to get a doctor just then and see what caused that. We could have received some immediate help. Instead, this is what happened. Roger got home, found me in the house, and told me what had happened to him. He was speaking just as normal as he always did, nothing at all indicating that he had a problem. Roger is very empathetic, so I said, "Oh, Roger, you were probably just so shook up seeing Jeff in that shape that you couldn't find the words you wanted to say." I really didn't think he had anything seriously wrong with him. I knew how easily he gets overwhelmed by sickness and diseases of other people (especially close friends and family). He almost can feel like he has the same things they have. I wanted to help him brush it off, so I said to him, "You need to quit thinking about Jeff right now. Get out in the yard and do some trimming of our bushes, etc., to put your mind on something else." Well, he went outside and went to work in the yard. That was Friday evening.

The next day, at some point, he went to write a check for something, and he came out from his office telling me that he couldn't write his name. I could not believe that, so I went into his office and asked him to write it, and he just could not write his name or anything else. Then I really did begin to get worried. I went on the Internet and looked up "Stroke Symptoms" and different tests you can give a person to check and see if they have had a stroke. I began immediately having Roger do all of these things that I had read, and he could do everything without a problem. That convinced me that it was not a stroke and that it would probably pass in time.

We made it through Saturday night. On Sunday morning, he was up and dressed for church when he came over to where I was fixing my hair at my vanity and sat down on a small settee beside the vanity.

He said, "Cherie, I know something is wrong. I think we should call 911 and get an ambulance to come and take me to a hospital downtown." He had already decided he wanted to be taken to Emory University Hospital. He knew that he should not be driving the way he felt, and I never drive on the interstates, especially to go downtown in Atlanta. Since it was Sunday morning and church time, we knew our family would all be in services right then. So, I did exactly that. I called 911 and Roger went out in the yard in his Sunday suit to wait on them to arrive.

When they pulled into our driveway with the siren blaring, a paramedic jumped out of the ambulance and said to Roger, "We had a call from here that someone may have had a stroke and needs to be carried to a hospital."

Roger quickly replied, "Yes, that's me!"

The paramedic then said, "Oh my God, man, you need to lie down. Let us get you on this stretcher." They then loaded him into the ambulance, and I rode up front with the driver, and off we went on our way to Emory's emergency room. During the ride, the paramedic who was with Roger in the back of the ambulance began to check him for stroke symptoms, like I had done the day before. He also told him that he really didn't think it was a stroke that he had. We happened to get to the ER door of the hospital at a perfect time, they were not busy, and there was no one ahead of us. They took him right in, ran a CT scan and a couple other tests, and the result they gave us was that he had indeed had a stroke. They told us about the damage they had seen to his brain cells. The doctor then told us that besides the present stroke, his brain also showed evidence of other strokes that had occurred at other times in the past, but they had no idea how long ago. I have wondered since then if maybe the time he had the extreme hearing loss and tinnitus in May could have been a stroke that really wreaked havoc on his ears.

They admitted him into the hospital. He was kept several days, and they did more testing, and his final diagnosis was called "acute aphasia" as a result of the stroke. He was released and sent to therapy for treatment each week to see the extent his brain had been damaged. He actually did quite well in therapy, and he was released after about seven weeks. We kept waiting for things to completely return to 100 percent normalcy as we had been told by our doctor that usually within a couple of years that can happen.

Several things did return quite soon. He had a very little amount of numbness on his right side which came back to normal after a time. His handwriting did not come back as quickly, and the thing that seems to be plaguing him the most is that his speech and word processing have not returned to the point that he can completely express his thoughts. Also, many times he will say a word that is directly opposite of the word he means. This is not only troubling and confusing and frustrating to him, but it is also difficult for us as we try to figure out exactly what he is meaning to say.

His stroke took place the end of October 2015. I am now writing this part of my book in the summer of 2018, and he has asked to once again go back to a speech pathologist and therapist. He wants to see if there is any more help that can be given so that he can get better use of the abilities he has lost in order to be able to make public presentations of our mission work in Albania. He also loved to preach whenever he got a chance. So that stroke made the second thing that was "his life's work" be put on hold, or go away permanently, we don't know yet.

We are adjusting as well as possible to the "new normal" for Roger and for me as his caregiver. I have watched him go through much depression over both losses. He has had to adjust to a much quieter lifestyle, and our travels have nearly ceased completely. We still go once a year to Albania to encourage our staff and love on the children. We meet with them on Skype on our computer all through the year for important business decisions, etc.

Muddy Water Boys

Roger says often, "I used to be an extrovert, but now I'm an introvert." This residual damage to Roger's ears and his speech process is very sad for me to see as his wife of fifty-seven years. I have been his partner in ministry all of our married lives. I was there to assist in all of the music in our family. We also had a musical group going in our senior years. We put together a group of men from our church and jokingly called them "The Muddy Water Boys." And the name stuck! That's what people called them, and they began to get quite a following, believe it or not! It was made up of Larry Alberts, Bob Loftin, Rick Smith, and Roger. They had actually been singing for a few years and were sounding good enough that they would get invited out to other churches to put on programs for their senior adults.

Those Muddy Water Boys were having such a great time. We all enjoyed their practice times, and it created a lot of fun and fellowship among the four couples. Bob's wife, Judi, also has a lot of musical ability, and she came to all the practices to help me sort out the parts for the guys as she has a great ear for harmony. Sometimes Larry's wife, Sue, would sit in on the practice times as she and Larry also worked together twenty-four seven for our church as professional caretakers for shut-ins, the hospitalized, and the bereaved. Judi and Sue and I love to sing, too, and we were threatening to form a ladies trio, but there never seemed to be any time left or "energy" after the guys would finish with their two- or three-hour practice. Rick's wife, Kathy, worked at a job away from home every day, so we didn't get to see her as much. However, we would get together socially on occasion and have a party. Kathy was then on hand to enter in and enjoy those festivities.

Rick and Roger were both sort of natural-born comedians, so whenever The Muddy Water Boys went to put on a full concert, they would throw in some of their comedy routines or impressions. Rick did a really good Elvis, and he was about the size of Elvis in his later years. That always went over really well. They actually sang one or two of Elvis's gospel songs at times. Really, when it came right down to it, all four of them were comedians. We sure laughed a lot at practices. In fact, we laughed nearly as much as they sang. I failed to put in that I was their pianist and their "director" at the practices. I made sure each person knew his part and stayed on it as much as humanly possible. I cracked a loud whip at times! They really made a lot of fun of me, but I have tough skin, so we just kept on as long as we possibly could, until Roger had these issues take him away. The Muddy Water Boys have never regrouped with anyone to take his place. We will always love this group of people, and we look back on our time together as a very special season in our lives.

Our family always loves to get together at least once a year to present a musical program. Sometimes, it's all Christian music, and sometimes, we have done Christmas concerts together. This includes everyone. Our kids, Buddy and Cindy, who are both married. Buddy's wife, Kerri, along with Cindy's two boys, Brady and Austin, and Buddy and Kerri's two girls, Victoria and Olivia. It has been the custom every year in October for our church, Glen Haven Baptist, to have "Hope for the World Sunday." On the evening of that date, we usually put together a family concert and are sometimes joined by the choir or special groups at our church. Roger has had to sit this out the last couple of years, and I usually don't get into the singing anymore either. I'm there if they need me on the piano, though. Roger used to be well known for his singing. He has recorded many solos through the years on over forty projects our family has recorded. As I stated earlier, he also had some good humorous songs and did a lot of funny things like dressing up as an old, old "country bumpkin" wearing his "bubba teeth" and singing "Wore Out." Many of you reading this book have seen him perform some of these songs. He loved nothing better than to make people laugh. If you asked me what I miss the most now, I'd have to say *Roger's humor*. He could always get a laugh out of me, and that has been a great thing that has kept us sane while going through all of these disabilities. We find something fun about it and laugh. Every once in a while, I'll bring up one of his old jokes that he has forgotten, and we'll have a new laugh all over again. We are both getting so old, I assure him, that we aren't really missing out on much because who in the world would want us to come and sing and joke for them now that we are this old?

I am feverishly working to complete my book before my eightieth birthday this month. My daughter, Cindy, and her husband, Andy, have planned on having a party for me along with their two sons, Brady and Austin, who also have birthdays in July. We always celebrate together. This year, however, I'll have very special guests at my birthday, my sisters and my brother. One of my sisters, Dolly, is coming from Granville Summit, Pennsylvania. Another sister, Trudy, is coming from Phoenix, Arizona. Patti will come from Chandler, Indiana, and Tom and his wife, Dolores, will drive over from Alabama. Some have not seen one another for at least ten years. How much fun we plan to have! I really do hope I get my book completed and published before I get any older and forget that I wrote it!

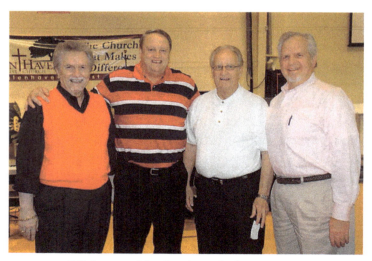

We became like family with these guys...
We spent hours practicing every week. Roger,
Rick Smith, Larry Alberts and Bob Loftin

Hope for the World Community Church Becomes a Reality

A few pages back, I mentioned that we were getting ready to open a church on our property in Marikaj, Albania, where the Hope Center is located. We had been praying for some time for the Lord to send us just the right person to pastor this new church plant. It seemed to be the desire of our Albanian staff to have an American pastor because that is what they were used to. It was American missionaries who planted some of the very first Bible-believing churches in Albania after the fall of communism. I suppose for that reason, the people there seem to think they are the best. In the last couple of years, we have been having some wonderful outreach events to not only the children of our community through the Saturday morning Kids Bible Club, and on Tuesday evening Teens Bible Study, but we have also held a number of special meetings around holidays and special days in Albania honoring mothers, teachers, etc. We have also held some amazing Vacation Bible School weeks there on the property.

Our own staff has been planning and preparing all of these events. However, an American missionary/pastor, Mike Fiocchi, has been involved much of the time. He had been pastoring a great church in Tirana and had led it to the point where they could have an Albanian pastor. That church has been under the leadership of the Albanian pastor for some time now, and Pastor Mike has begun to work in another location, planting another church in a village not too far from Tirana. This work is fairly new, probably two years old or so. He has always been happy to come and preach at some of the special meetings we have had at the Hope Center in Marikaj. The people from the community who attended those services liked him very much. Of course, our staff there has known him for years, and some of them attend the church in Tirana where he was pastor for a good while. Well, I'm not sure how it came to be, but our HFTW president, Perparim Demcellari, began to talk with Mike about our need for a pastor in order to get the church established there in Marikaj. He knew Mike had a new work on Sundays in another village, but he asked him if he thought he might begin the church there in Marikaj with services being held on Saturday rather than Sunday. Pastor Mike apparently liked this idea and said he would pray about it and see if God would lead him to do that.

Well, we were so blessed when we heard that he was willing, and felt led of the Lord, to come and pastor this new church. He checked with his mission board to be sure they had no problem with him doing this, and God made a way for us to finally open up the church for which we had been praying for so long. It will be called "Hope for the World Community Church." It will be open to the surrounding community. Our staff at the Hope Center, as well as our teens, will be very active in this new church. They have worked so hard in planting the "Gospel seeds" for the church. They have established a very good reputation in the community to where people who were first skeptical of what Hope for the World was doing there on that property have come to trust us with their precious children in weekly Bible studies and many other Christian events. We have been so thrilled to see not only the young people coming to our property during the past couple of years, but also adults have frequented the premises for various gatherings celebrating Christmas, Easter, Mother's Day, Teacher's Day, etc. Our president, Perparim Demcellari, has also held many meetings where he invited the older men of the community to come and enjoy fellowship, discuss Bible topics, and, at times, hear a testimony from someone special. All of these things have been allowing us to plant the seeds to establish a church at the Hope Center. It has been an amazing thing to watch. The church has been growing with people even before we had a pastor or an official name for the church.

At many of these events and Bible Studies for Teens, Pastor Mike Fiocchi had been the one bringing the Word of God to the various groups. They have all enjoyed him very much, and hearts have been touched and knit together through his ministry on these occasions. As I mentioned earlier, our weekly service will be on Saturday instead of Sunday, at least temporarily. This is because Pastor Mike's other new church meets on Sunday. Pastor Mike has agreed to come and help us get it started and to be the interim pastor until God calls someone else to do so full-time. We are just trusting God in all of this and asking for his divine will. We could not be any more pleased as Pastor Mike has built a very strong church in Tirana which is now pastored by one of the Albanian pastors who was called to preach under his ministry. Pastor Mike, his wife, Jennifer, and their children, have been in Albania a good number of years. I believe it has been at least twenty years. We have known him all of those years, so we know he is a wonderful man of God and a great pastor. He also has a good command of the Albanian language which is a tremendous blessing. Their daughter is also a great pianist and will be playing for the services, and his son will be our worship leader for the musical part of the service. You can see that God has truly provided just what we need. Our staff and teens, who are a part of the Hope Center, will be very involved in the church. We are looking forward to seeing each of them taking an active role in reaching the community and also in helping each week with the children's classes that will continue to meet just prior to the church service.

We are using our gym on the property as the main auditorium for church. It will continue to be multifunctional both as a gym for the kids during the week and as a church on the weekend. We will continue having the kids Bible class each Saturday morning at the Hope Center, and then it will flow right into the worship service. That way, all the kids who come for Bible class can stay for church. We are hoping to reach their parents, too, as they have come to know us and trust us with their children. The religious background of the community is Muslim. However, not many people in Albania are actually practicing Islam. They, too, had been completely shut down during the years of the communist dictatorship. So, in reality, the doors did not open for *any* religious teaching in Albania until 1992, after having been totally closed for around fifty years or more, under the communistic and atheistic regime.

We thank the Lord for their openness to the Gospel since 1992. There are many good Christian ministries in Albania now. There are good Bible-teaching churches in many different places in the country. We have seen a tremendous growth in the outreach of the Gospel during the twenty-five years that we have been coming to Albania. We have been allowed to teach the Bible in each of the government orphanages with which we have been connected all during this time. We have seen great changes in the lives of the boys and girls through the years as well. This is not only obvious to us, but it has been obvious to the government directors, workers, and even to the mayors of the cities and directors and staff of social services. We have received many certificates of gratitude through the years from the cities where we have been working with not only the children but also with the elderly center in Saranda, Albania.

We are so happy that our church is opening now because Roger and I are not getting any younger, and this is a dream we have had for a number of years and it is finally coming to fruition. We pray that this will be a great church that will bring many, many people to the Lord. Our lives during these years have been so blessed because of the many ways we have seen God working in the lives of the people of Albania under the leadership of Hope for the World. To God be the glory! Great things *he* has done!

And now, I am coming toward the end of this particular book. It has been a joy to reflect on the past twenty-five years of our lives in this way. It has taken me about four years to complete this one. I am so happy to have had the help of so many wonderful friends who were willing to insert their own personal testimonies and stories into this book.

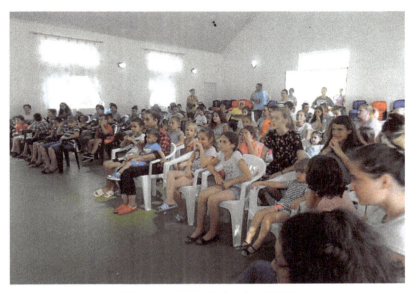

Vacation Bible School—2018
Closing Ceremony Crowd.

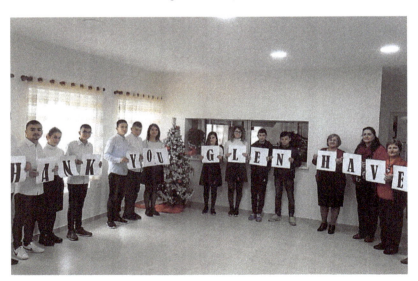

Beautiful Dining Hall completed with special offerings From Glen Haven
Baptist Church, McDonough, GA
(Our Home Church), plus another very, very special friend.

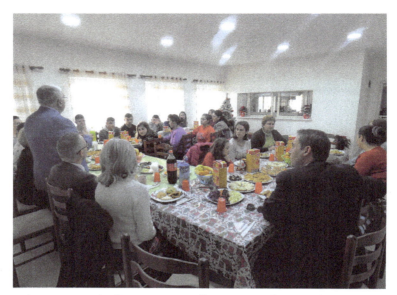

A great crowd of our teens, staff, Pastors Mike Fiocchi and Ari and families gathered in our new dining hall on Christmas Day at the Hope Center. First meal in this beautiful new restoration.

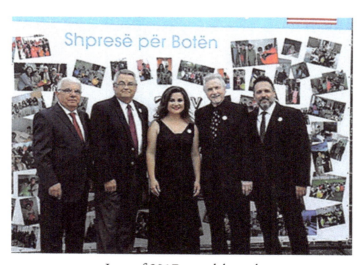

June of 2017 we celebrated
25 Years in Albania as Hope for the World Foundation
Perparim Demcellari, Jimmy Franks, Ledina
Rabdishta, Roger Mullins and Buddy Mullins

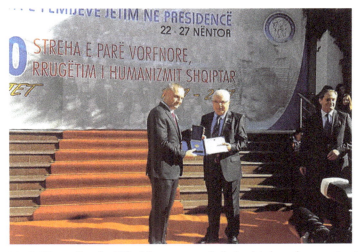

In 2018 Hope for the World was awarded the highest humanitarian award from the country of Albania. Pictured is President llir Meta presenting The Mother Theresa Award and Medallion to our HFTW Albanian President—Perparim Demcellari

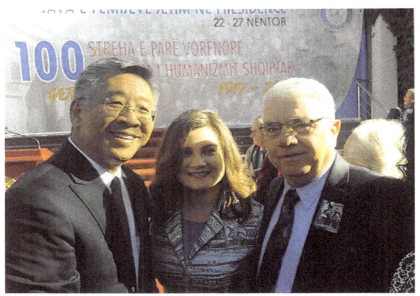

Also present to congratulate HFTW was
The United States Ambassador, Donald Lu.
Picitured, Ambassador Lu, Ledina and Perparim.

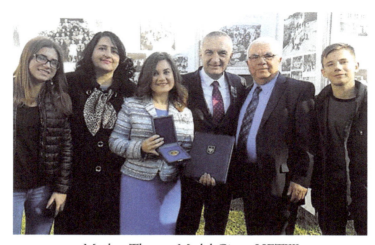

Mother Theresa Medal Given HFTW
In this Photo—President of Albania—Ilir Meta
And HFTW President Perparim Demcellari with Ledina
Rabdishta, Margarita Gjoni and two of
Our teens from the Hope Center. A Very
Memorable occasion for all of them.

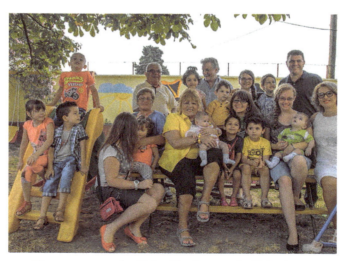

Here we are at the Baby Orphanage in Shkodra…
So many babies have come and gone from this
Orphanage since we started there in 1992. Many have been
adopted through the years. But all have heard about Jesus.

THE MAKING OF A WONDERFUL LIFE

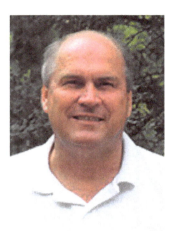

Chris Martin—Friend and Project Leader
Chris has brought many, many work groups into Albania to work—mainly to Saranda Orphanage. We are so thankful for him. He is still doing this currently. Thankful for him.

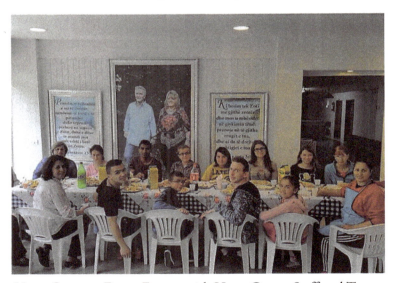

Hope Center—Easter Feast—with Hope Center Staff and Teens.
They insisted on putting this "larger-than-life"
photo of us on the wall to make it like we
are there in person at all these gatherings.

Come with Us

Our foundation is highly respected and well known in Albania as we have been helping these orphans since 1992, right after the communist wall finally fell in that country. Everyone who goes with us always tells us they feel like it is more of a vacation than a "mission trip." We have *such a great time!*

Dress is casual. We usually go in either May or September, so the weather is perfect! Bermuda-length shorts are fine to wear. A light jacket may be needed in the evening in some places. We will go to church on Sunday, so a skirt or dress is advisable for the ladies.

All expenses are paid up front to our organization, and our staff takes care of handling expenses and tipping at all of the restaurants and hotels. We will be staying in four different cities in Albania and one city on the island of Corfu, Greece, before coming home. *All of this is included in the "Tour of Orphanages" trip.*

If you would like to know more about Albania, and their customs and culture, I have also prepared an orientation manual and a language guide to assist each member of our tour groups. Albania has its own language called Shqip (pronounced "Ship"). We will have interpreters with us at all times, and many Albanians know "some" English. Most all of our staff members speak English fluently. If you have any other specific questions, please do not hesitate to ask us. You may do so by going to our website, www.hopefortheworldalbania.com, and sending us an inquiry from there. You will see various types of missions described. If you do not want to tour with us, but instead prefer to go on a work mission, or a summer mission, all of that is addressed on our beautiful website. *If you prefer to email us or call us and discuss this, feel free to do so.*

Our email: RogMullins@charter.net; *Phone:* 1-888-212-HOPE (4673)

God has truly been good to us all of these years we have been ministering in Albania, and we are by no means finished yet. We may be old, but we are not dead! As of the time of the writing of this book, which is in 2018, Roger is seventy-seven, and I am eighty, but we still carry the full load of responsibility for the work in Albania. We have a wonderful staff, most of whom you have met in this book. They do the hands-on ministry in Albania with the orphans, widows, and handicapped. Through our special projects ministries, "Hands of Hope," they reach many, many more groups and individuals.

We have quite a budget to meet each month, and it is met by the gifts of God's people who feel a burden to help us. Some do so by sponsoring a child, while others contribute to the general fund of Hope for the World Albania. We are thankful for those who contribute as "Torchbearers" to support us personally, as this is our only source of income. We do not take funds for our personal needs from those sent in for the ministry but churches and individuals who have expressed a desire to contribute to us personally do this monthly. Everyone's giving record is kept very carefully, and all gifts are fully tax deductible.

I have no way of knowing how much longer Roger and I will be able to continue with our part in Albania, but I do know that we have things in place, and people in place, to continue the work when we can no longer do it. Our son, Buddy, and his wife, Kerri, and our daughter, Cindy, all know the workings of our office fully. Cindy has worked with us for many years. They all have been several times to Albania and know all of our wonderful people over there so that they can continue to build and grow this work in future years.

We are trusting the Lord to take good care of this ministry in Albania, and we believe the scripture that says in Philippians 1:6:

> Being confident of this very thing, that he which hath begun a good work in you will perform it until the day of Jesus Christ.

We praise the Lord for this wonderful *Albanian Attachment* He has given us for so many, many years!

Epilogue
Israel

As I have been writing *The Albanian Attachment*, many thoughts have prompted me to add another chapter in our lives concerning travel that was not mission-related travel. In my last book, I chose to write the epilogue about our one and only mission trip to Romania. There is something very endearing to me about traveling to foreign countries. I am always intrigued by the different cultures, people, food, customs, architecture, flowers, animals, and even the terrain of the country. That being said, I am going to take some time now to share with you my favorite place on earth to visit—Israel, "The Holy Land."

We were serving on the church staff at Madisonville Baptist Temple in 1975 when our pastor, Bob Lamb, gathered a group of people together to take a ten-day Holy Land tour. Roger was the youth director at the church at that time, and I was Pastor Lamb's secretary. As the time drew closer for the trip, something came up on our pastor's schedule that was suddenly making it impossible for him to host the group. His way was already paid, so he asked Roger if he would like to take his place and host the tour to Israel.

Well, gee whiz, who wouldn't want to go to Israel? He didn't have places for two people to go because his wife, Willa, had not planned to go in the first place. That meant that Roger could go, but I could not. That was OK with me because we had our two kids who were ages seven and eleven at that time, and I really needed to stay home with them. So as it happened, Roger was excited to go in Brother Bob's place, and I was happy for him as he had never been to Israel before and, in fact, had not been doing much international travel, if any, since we had been married. Probably his last travel overseas had been in the military.

The time came for the trip. I had gotten Roger's things together for him and his suitcase packed. We were very happy that he had this opportunity, even though he had absolutely no knowledge about hosting a group of people on a tour of any type. Nothing like on-the-job training! We lived in Madisonville, Kentucky, but his trip originated from Louisville, Kentucky, where he had a number of travelers joining him. I really don't remember how many there were in that group, but I can remember seeing a photo of them in Israel, and I would guess there were somewhere between thirty and forty in the group.

When Roger got to Israel and met the tour guide, Motti, he felt like he had met a lifelong friend. Motti had such an awesome personality and loved to joke around a lot. He and Roger were nearly the same age, with similar builds, and both had dark curly hair. If you were just looking at them, you might think they were blood brothers. Motti was a "professional tour guide for Holyland Pilgrimage Tours," and Roger knew immediately that they were in great hands with Motti leading them around Israel.

Motti not only became an instant friend to Roger but also bonded with a couple from Louisville, Kentucky, David and Freda Parker. This was their first trip to Israel, and they had brought along other friends and family members. They all really took to Motti. They were older than Roger and Motti, but this became for them the beginning of many years of visiting the Holy Land and a lifelong connection to the entire Kalmovitcz family. Motti's wife's name is Aviva. She did not take the tours with the groups, but through the years, it became customary that Aviva would meet up with the Parkers and Roger or "us" at some point during the days spent in Jerusalem.

Motti and Aviva had two daughters and a son. Their son was named Ezer, or Ezra, and he was the cutest curly haired big-eyed little guy back then! We have been told by Ezer himself that through the years, the Parker family would invite them to their home in Kentucky, and Ezer was taught by Dave Parker how to drive a tractor on his farm. This was a great thing for him because he grew up in the city of Jerusalem and had absolutely no experience with farm life. I understand this became something that Ezer so loved and looked forward to throughout his childhood. I have heard that the families would even swap houses at times. Motti and his family would come and live in the Parker's home in Kentucky while Dave and Freda would go and live in their home in Jerusalem. We were busy traveling on the road in our evangelism ministry as a family during the years between 1977 and 1994. Our only home was our bus, so we couldn't host people visiting in America during much of that time. I do recall, however, once when Motti was in America, we took him with us in our "Home on Wheels" for a short trip to Indiana. We held a Sunday afternoon concert at Good Shepherd Baptist Church near Indianapolis. Motti came that day and gave a little talk about the Holy Land, helping us to prepare for the next Israel trip as Roger and I continued to host Holy Land tours as often as we could. We had a good way of promoting them since we traveled most of the time. Many people from the churches where we ministered went with us. We treasure those times!

By then, I had been able to join Roger for these tours, and I was just as much mesmerized by the country as he was, and I certainly had fallen in love with Motti and Aviva! We would get our pictures taken with them whenever we were with them. She was such a cute little lady! I remember getting to meet their kids one time when they were all pretty young. One of the girls was in the military when we saw her. In Israel, every young person, boys and girls, has to serve time in the Israeli Army when they graduate from high school. Their country really instills patriotism in them during that time, if it had not already been embedded in them by their parents.

Having this wonderful friendship with Motti and Aviva and their kids has made us feel so much a part of Israel through the years. We feel like we have "family" over there. At the time I am writing, Roger has estimated that he has made fifteen or more trips to Israel through the years. Oh, how I wish I had kept track of each trip and the people who went with us! Why is it I can keep such good records for all of my work pertaining to Albania, but when it comes to Israel and our tours over there, when the tour ended, I just let the records go except for pictures I took while we were in the country.

For a number of years, in the mid-1990s and early 2000s, we did not take any trips to Israel, but in 2010, we began having some of our pastor friends contact us and ask us if we would be willing to plan another trip to the Holyland Pilgrimage Tours. Roger said that he would definitely love to do that if he could still have Motti to go with us as our guide. We had not talked to Motti for years, so I really didn't know if he was still working for Holy Land tours. He said to me one day in 2009, "Cherie, look here, I still have this business card of Motti's. I'm gonna try to give him a call in Jerusalem." He picked up the phone here in our Hope for the World office and dialed Motti's number, and, lo and behold, Motti answered the phone! How awesome was that? What an amazing conversation they had reminiscing and catching up on the years we had not been in touch. How in the world had we let so many years slip past since our last trip?

Well, plans were made right away with Motti for another visit to Israel with a group in 2010. We began letting friends know that we were going again after so many years. We had pastor friends and their wives from different states go with us. We knew that this was going to be a wonderful trip and a reunion with Motti. We were all grandparents now as our children were grown and married, even Motti's son, little Ezer. When we got to Israel, we found out that Ezer was getting very involved in the tour business, too. In fact, he came along one day, and Motti let him give us the lecture on the model of the "Old City" during the days of Jesus. He did an awesome job, and we could see that he had learned from the very best.

We took our son, Buddy, with us so he could furnish our group with some great music along the way. He and Ezer really hit it off, and it was great to see that friendship developing as Roger's and Motti's relationship had been so close for so many years. They were like brothers, just from different sides of the water. That is what we are seeing now with Ezer and Buddy as they are working together today on Holy Land tours now that Roger and I have sort of "retired" from taking groups.

THE MAKING OF A WONDERFUL LIFE

We were invited over to Motti's and Aviva's home one day for lunch. It was such a blessing to see the nice home that they had and to see how God had prospered Motti through the years. Aviva was the superintendent or administrator of one of the largest hospitals, if not *the* largest one in Jerusalem. We saw their daughters and their grandchildren and learned about their lives. It was such a wonderful time we had there "catching up" over the many years that we had missed one another.

I failed to tell you that when I got to Israel and saw Motti, instead of him *working* for Holyland Pilgrimage Tours, we found that he now *owned* the company! What a wonderful blessing! It also made us much more appreciative of him still being willing to tour us all over Israel.

Motti had such a wonderful personality and was so humorous along with it. He would have all of us laughing on the bus as we toured from site to site in Israel. He loved our singing, and he knew so many of our songs and hymns that he would often request certain songs. He had a word that he had coined, and he used it in many ways when he was describing someone or really talking down on anyone he happened to dislike. He'd call them a "chickalaboomba." For instance, I remember once there were some road workers alongside the street who were supposed to be getting a job done, and he could see that most of them were doing nothing. He'd say, "Look at those lazy chickalaboombas!"

Oh, what a wonderful trip we had with Motti as he took us around from Caesarea by the sea to Tiberias and the Sea of Galilee. This is where we stayed in one of the most beautiful seaside resorts—Gai Beach. After dinner that first night, Motti was outside with us looking at the beautiful Sea of Galilee with the lights shining down from the mountain across the sea. He said to all of us, "Do you know what those lights are?" He asked Roger specifically, and because Roger had been there before, he assumed Roger should know.

When Roger told him, "No, Motti, I don't know what those lights are.".

Motti then said, "Why, they're Israelites!" And we all had a great laugh at that. You see what a great guy Motti was?

Our next day he took us across the Sea of Galilee on one of the boats. We had a wonderful service right in the middle of the sea. We had scriptures read about Jesus walking on the sea and bidding Peter to come and walk on the water. We all know that as long as Peter kept his eyes on Jesus, he was walking on top of the waves, but as soon as he took his eyes off of Christ, he began to sink, but Jesus caught him and picked him up and put him back on board.

While in that area, we got to visit a museum that housed a fishing boat that had been dug out from the sand that dated back to Jesus's day. It took a very special method to bring that up out of the water and sand so it would not deteriorate. We saw a video of that process. It was very interesting, and just to think we were looking at a boat from way back then was awesome!

We also had our son, Buddy, with us on our first return trip to Israel, so we always had some good music everywhere we went. In the next few years, we had Buddy and Kerri, and even our daughter, Cindy, and her husband, Andy. Some of our very closest friends and other family members have also been with us. In thinking about crossing the Sea of Galilee, I recall that when Cindy and Buddy were with us, we sang some of our old songs. One of them was "He's the Master of the Sea," written by our friend, Squire Parsons. We sang that song years ago when we traveled as a family, so it was fun to "resurrect" it and try to sing it right there on the beautiful Sea of Galilee. We always had a pastor in our group read from some of the Scriptures that took place on or around that beautiful place. We had some truly spirit-filled times!

The year we had Cindy and Andy with us we also had our niece, DeAnne Stumbo, and her husband, Scott, along. In fact, Roger married them just a few days before our trip, and so they actually spent their honeymoon in Israel. All in all, there were eight of our family members enjoying this trip to Israel together. What a time we had!

I also loved each time we would go to the Jordan River and have a baptismal service for any and all who wanted to be baptized in the Jordan River, the very river where John baptized Jesus at the beginning of his public ministry. I'll never forget these precious times! I usually held people's personal items for them while they were baptized. I've seen Roger and Buddy baptize a good number of people there, as well as other pastors in our group. This is truly a highlight of the trip.

Once we resumed our visits to Israel in 2010, we kept going back nearly every year. We have had the privilege to take our senior pastor, Stan Berrong, and his wife, Jacki, from our home church, Glen Haven Baptist of McDonough, Georgia, with us on one of those trips. Then the next year, we took another staff pastor, Mike Creasman, and his wife, Gwen, with us. They enjoyed it so much that they told us they wanted to go again sometime. Buddy hosted a trip in 2016 and took another staff pastor, Warren Green, and his wife, Jenny, on that trip. Pastor Stan and Jacki are planning to cohost a tour with Buddy and Kerri in March of 2019. It looks like that trip will be at least one hundred people in number.

In the month of February, for several years, we have had the privilege of having Motti and Ezer or Ezer and his mother, Aviva, visit in our home in Georgia. They have also been special guests at our church where they have promoted the next tour that we were hosting. I am so thankful that Motti came to be with us in one of those recent years, because it was during the following year that we received a phone call from him letting us know he had been very sick. I believe he told Roger he thought he had pneumonia, but it turned out that he had pancreatic cancer. He managed to work his tours right up until just a short time before he passed away. He was such a strong man and a great example to his son, Ezer. He was an amazing man and one of our very dearest friends. His life was a blessing to so many as he led us through Jerusalem and all over the Holy Land. He was so proud of his son, Ezer, and had taught him so much about the business that it was a perfect fit for Ezer to step right into Motti's shoes and provide the best of the best when it comes to guiding our tours over there.

Ezer is not only the owner of the tour business and greatest tour guide, but he also teaches the other tour guides in Jerusalem at the university. He tries to stress to them how important it is for them to not just give the facts, historically and biblically, but to also put their own heart and soul into sharing these wonderful truths with the people. Ezer does that! You know that he believes what he is telling you and that he has a personal relationship with the Christ, the Messiah! He is full of worship and praise and joins in with our singing everywhere we go in Israel. He, like his dad, has some favorite songs that he has learned from his many visitors from America.

The year 2015 was what we felt would be our last trip to Israel. Mainly because of my personal inability to make the long walks and sometimes difficult steps, etc. We had the trip scheduled for August, and we were cohosting it with Buddy and Kerri. We had planned this trip to be mainly managed by them as we wanted them to learn the ropes, so to speak, of planning and hosting tours to Israel. It had been such a blessing to us through the years to take so many people on the Holy Land Pilgrimage, and we hoped that they would continue this as a part of their ministry in years to come.

As the time drew closer and closer to our August departure date, Roger's anxiety and periods of depression, due to tinnitus in his ears, seemed to get worse and worse. He just didn't think he could even enjoy the tour and was thinking he would have to back out altogether and let Buddy and Kerri handle it on their own this time. I distinctly remember writing an email to Ezer telling him that we were going to have to cancel.

I also recall very vividly that I had just been to see the movie *The War Room* in a local theater with a group from our church. Roger couldn't go, as the sound in theaters really messed up his ears. I came home with a new determination to walk and pray all through my house and do war against the attack from Satan that we were under, particularly on Roger and his ears and emotions. I got up early one morning and spent a good while doing battle in prayer concerning Roger and asking the Lord to make a way for him to take this one last trip to Israel that was coming right up in the next day or two. When he came out of the bedroom that morning, I had prayer with him and I begged God to make a way so that we could go and to provide a calming for Roger's anxiety and the tinnitus that was tormenting him. Well, after that prayer, in just a matter of minutes, I got a phone call from a family member about something totally unrelated, but she asked me how he was doing. When I told her, she then told me that she had some pills that she thought would really help him in his distress.

She said, "I'll be right there and bring them for you to try." She did, and we did try them, and I want you to know, it was like a magic pill she had brought to him.

He called me into his office about a half hour after taking that pill and said, "You know what, I'm all better, and I believe I can go to Israel if I take some of these pills with me." We got some from his doctor, and Roger was able to make the trip with very little difficulty. It was amazing! I knew the Lord had heard my prayers, and that was the greatest thing!

This particular trip in August of 2015 is one we will never forget. We had a wonderful group of friends with us, many of them were from Buddy's church in Florida. One man in particular, Bob Lynch, was intensely videoing and photographing everything on that trip. We even laughed about it because we seldom saw his face out from behind a camera of some kind. Little did we know that we would later be presented with DVD's from him of the *entire tour*. He had fully edited the material and added some wonderful inspirational music (some of it from our family's recordings). God has provided us this wonderful memory of that trip that will forever be very special to us since we went there feeling that it would be our last time to go.

I recall a very special blessing when we were in Israel and actually gathered on the site of the synagogue in Capernaum where Jesus frequented and taught on so many occasions. Much of the building is still standing. One of the men on the tour asked to have the men gather around Roger and put their hands on him and pray over him because of what he had been suffering. It was a very, very special time of prayer and asking the Lord to calm the anxiety it had caused him. It was a wonderful time of prayer and expectation there on that actual property where Jesus had ministered during his years on earth. We will never forget that experience.

When we are visiting the various sites in Israel, there is something very special about each place we visit. There is no way for me to express in writing the feelings you get while traveling over the land where Jesus walked and talked and performed miracles. Where he was born and grew up, was baptized, and then preached. We walked where he taught his disciples and broke bread with them in the upper room just before he was betrayed by Judas. We also visited the ruins of Peter's mother-in-law's home where Jesus stayed while in Capernaum. It has been nearly completely excavated, and it is amazing to see. We loved walking over the many places from the Bible where miracles were performed. What a precious time we spent in prayer and worship and praise at the Mount of Beatitudes where we could see the place where Christ fed the five thousand men plus women and children. Oh, so many wonderful experiences we had!

Probably one of the favorite spots was on the Mount of Olives, looking over at the Eastern Gate of the old city that has been blocked for ages. One day, Jesus will return and come through that Eastern Gate! Praise the Lord! The Garden of Gethsemane is another favorite place. We saw the ancient olive trees still growing there that date back to Jesus's day. Perhaps we even saw the one under which he knelt and prayed. We have had some very heart-touching times of worship and praise there in that Garden. Ezer even arranged for us to be in there in a very special section of the Garden. One time the guards of the Garden forgot we were in there and went off and locked us in. What a place to be a prisoner! We had a great laugh about that, but we weren't detained too long, and we loved every extra minute we had.

When in Jerusalem, we walked in Jesus's footsteps down beneath the city streets of Old Jerusalem to the Praetorium, the actual place where Jesus was scourged by the Roman soldiers until his flesh hung from him. It's also the place where those same soldiers gambled over his garments at the time of his crucifixion. It is the exact place. We saw the stones where the soldiers gambled for his robe. We stood right where he was when he bore the stripes by which we are healed.

We could see the diagrams of the gambling games in the stone floor and even blood stains were on the stones that were no doubt made by the blood of Jesus. This is truly a place where we felt we were standing on "Holy Ground," as this is literally the exact spot where Jesus's torture took place. It is not within the proximity, it is the *actual place*. Ezer is always careful to let us know if we are approximately at a place where Christ was or actually on the very historically proven place. Such is the case with the Praetorium. I'm so glad I have personally been there a number of times in my life to experience worship. I can't praise him enough for dying for my sins. What a great experience to be there singing with fellow Christians, "We are Standing on Holy Ground."

There is nothing like the final day of a tour in Jerusalem when we get to visit Golgotha's Hill and sit where we can look right at the mountain called "Golgotha," the "place of the skull." It is a very distinct impression in the ancient rock that resembles a skull. It is just outside the gates of the city, as written in the Scriptures. It is at Gordon's Tomb, and it seems to be the place where Jesus was crucified because right next to it is a beautiful garden that has been there for thousands of years. There's a place where you can look below to a lower level of the garden where they had a water system that dates back to the days of Christ and indicates this was the garden of a very wealthy person, no doubt. It was their method of keeping the garden watered. This is the Garden Tomb where Jesus was buried. It is so easy to read the scriptures and then look at this setting and truly believe you are in the exact location where it took place.

We not only got to look at the tomb, but we each got to go inside of the tomb and see the place where they had laid our Savior. They have made a door for the entrance now that can be closed, but you can see the trough for the huge rock that was rolled across the entrance back then. There are other tombs like that in the country that we saw in our travels that show how they were made. The rock is like a huge solid wheel in a track that could be pushed by several men to make it roll across the tomb's entrance. One person, however, would never be able to move it alone. That is just another indication of the miracle concerning Christ's resurrection, the actual rolling away of that great stone from the opening of the tomb.

When we entered the tomb, I could truly sense the Holy Spirit's presence. Only about four people at a time can go in. We cannot touch the place where his body laid but just look through a man-made fence that separates us from the rest of the tomb. You can, however, see just how his body would have fit right there in that very special place. I'm so thankful I have been there, even though I believed before I ever went.

On the man-made door on the inside of the tomb, they have a wonderful sign which reads, "He is Not Here, He is Risen." This is shouting ground! It is because of our resurrected Lord and Savior that we, too, can have eternal life. Christianity is the only religion whose leader has arisen from the dead. Historically, they have never ever been able to find the remains of Christ after he was crucified. He arose! He arose! Hallelujah, Christ arose!

I don't know if I will ever get to go back to Israel during my remaining time on earth, but I can certainly say I will look forward to going there again when Christ rules and reigns from the throne of David during the millennium or during the endless ages of eternity when we as Christians are all together with him. Some of my friends who aren't able to go to Israel have said, "I'll just wait and go with the original cast."

Of all the places I have been in this life, I am *most* anxious to get to heaven one day. I have so many family members and loved ones there already waiting on me. Just knowing that I will get to look on my Savior's face and thank him personally for saving my soul as a young teenaged girl by my mother's bedside in Harpursville, New York, on a Friday night in March of 1954, will be so worth it all! That is my "born-again birthday." I can't wait to get to heaven one day to thank Jesus personally and then experience eternal life with him and all of the saints from Genesis to Revelation. I thank God for my godly heritage and for so many Christian family members and friends I have here on earth. I will look so forward to seeing all of them when I get there. I hope you are planning to be there, too.

In conclusion to this epilogue, let me tell you that I just finished reading an awesome book by David Jeremiah entitled *The Agents of the Apocalypse*. I'd like to use some of the words taken from the last few pages in his book.

> *All people are born with an unquenchable thirst in their lives that can only be filled with Jesus, the "water of life", spoken of in the book of Revelation*

22:17 by John. They try to satisfy that thirst with things of the world, such as pleasure, accomplishments, possessions, relationships or power, but in time they find that these things do not satisfy. Even Solomon said, after trying wealth, sex, power and glory, "It is vanity, vanity vanity." (Or, as my father used to explain it when he was preaching, it is like "soap bubbles, soap bubbles, soap bubbles.")

When you realize that nothing on earth will satisfy your longing, or "thirst", that is when you are close to coming to know Christ. The God-shaped vacuum in your life can only be filled by God, the Creator, made known in the flesh as Jesus Christ. If you have not taken a drink of that water, I urge you to do so now, while you still have breath. The Bible says in Romans 10:13, 'Whoever calls on the name of the LORD shall be saved.' I hope you'll call upon Him and quench your thirst now and forever.

May God bless you and your family,
Cherie

Notes:
Epilogue:
Adapted from David Jeremiah, *The Agents of the Apocalypse: A Riveting Look at the Key Players of the End Times.*
Copyright 2014 by David Jeremiah. All rights reserved.
Published in association with Yates & Yates (www.yates2.com)
Tyndale Publishers

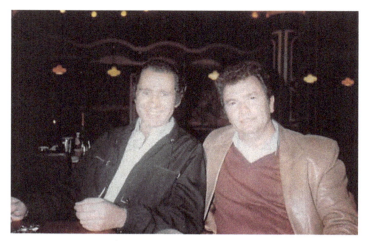

Motti and Roger back in the 70's when they began their lifetime friendship and Israel tours Together with Holy Land Pilgrimage Tours.

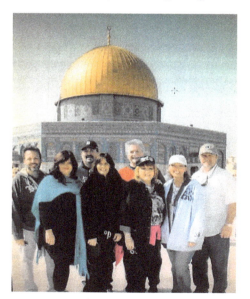

Family in Israel—2013
We were blessed to have our son Buddy and his wife Kerri, our Niece, Deanne and her husband Scott, and Our daughter, Cindy and her husband, Andy with us In Israel this time. A wonderful experience!

THE MAKING OF A WONDERFUL LIFE

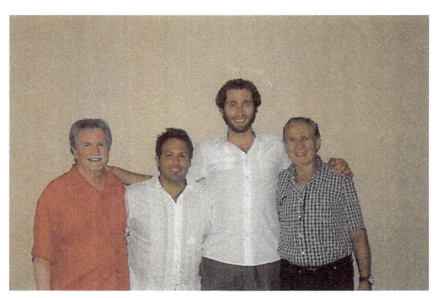

"Like Father, Like Son"…
Roger, Buddy, Ezer and Motti (Father, son, Father, son)
Ezer continues the Family Business since
His father passed. Holyland Pilgrimage Tours.
Buddy continues hosting tours in our place.
This has been going on since 1978…
Amazing and Awesome Relationship…
Truly added to our Wonderful Life

About the Author

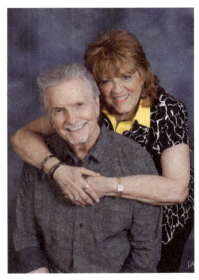

Me and my husband... Roger and Cherie Mullins

Cherie Y. Mullins is the wife of Evangelist Roger Mullins. She is the daughter of the late Leo and Beverly Forse, of Binghamton, New York. As she grew up, they were members of the well-known Little White Church of Conklin, New York. Her family and church foundations play a tremendous role in her life of ministry with her husband today. As a couple, they have served the Lord faithfully in full-time evangelism, Christian music, and missionary work since 1969. They reside in McDonough, Georgia, and are members of Glen Haven Baptist Church. The family has traveled in evangelism and gospel music from 1978 to 1994. The family has recorded forty gospel music projects which include a piano solo

CD by Cherie. Today, she works daily in the offices of Hope for the World Albania with her husband, Roger, and their daughter, Cindy.

Since 1994, they have been ministering to thousands of orphan children of Albania, hundreds of senior citizens, and many who are both physically and mentally challenged, through Hope for the World, as directors of this ministry. Their son, Buddy Mullins, is currently the CEO of the Hope for the World Foundation ministering in six different countries.

CPSIA information can be obtained
at www.ICGtesting.com
Printed in the USA
LVHW071631210323
742160LV00012B/885